Equine Urinary Tract Disorders

Editor

THOMAS J. DIVERS

VETERINARY CLINICS OF NORTH AMERICA: EQUINE PRACTICE

www.vetequine.theclinics.com

April 2022 • Volume 38 • Number 1

ELSEVIER

1600 John F. Kennedy Boulevard • Suite 1800 • Philadelphia, Pennsylvania, 19103-2899

http://www.vetequine.theclinics.com

VETERINARY CLINICS OF NORTH AMERICA: EQUINE PRACTICE Volume 38, Number 1
April 2022 ISSN 0749-0739, ISBN-13: 978-0-323-81351-8

Editor: Katerina Heidhausen
Developmental Editor: Ann Gielou Posedio

Veterinary Clinics of North America: Equine Practice (ISSN 0749-0739) is published in April, August, and December by Elsevier Inc., 360 Park Avenue South, New York, NY 10010-1710. Business and Editorial Offices: 1600 John F. Kennedy Blvd., Suite 1800, Philadelphia, PA 19103-2899. Subscription prices are $299.00 per year (domestic individuals), $777.00 per year (domestic institutions), $100.00 per year (domestic students/residents), $341.00 per year (Canadian individuals), $789.00 per year (Canadian institutions), $372.00 per year (international individuals), $789.00 per year (international institutions), $100.00 per year (Canadian students/residents), and $180.00 per year (international students/residents). To receive student/resident rate, orders must be accompanied by name of affiliated institution, date of term, and the signature of program/residency coordinator on institution letterhead. Orders will be billed at individual rate until proof of status is received. Foreign air speed delivery is included in all *Clinics* subscription prices. All prices are subject to change without notice. **POSTMASTER:** Send address changes to *Veterinary Clinics of North America: Equine Practice*, 3251 Riverport Lane, Maryland Heights, MO 63043. Customer Service (orders, claims, online, change of address): Elsevier Health Sciences Division, Subscription **Customer Service, 3251 Riverport Lane, Maryland Heights, MO 63043. Tel: 1-800-654-2452 (U.S. and Canada); 314-447-8871 (outside U.S. and Canada). Fax: 314-447-8029. E-mail: journalscustomerservice-usa@elsevier.com (for print support);** E-mail: journalsonlinesupport-usa@ elsevier.com (for online support).

Reprints. For copies of 100 or more of articles in this publication, please contact the Commercial Reprints Department, Elsevier Inc., 360 Park Avenue South, New York, NY 10010-1710. Tel.: 212-633-3874; Fax: 212-633-3820; E-mail: reprints@elsevier.com.

Veterinary Clinics of North America: Equine Practice is covered in *MEDLINE/PubMed (Index Medicus), Excerpta Medica, Current Contents/Agriculture, Biology and Environmental Sciences, and ISI.*

Contributors

EDITOR

THOMAS J. DIVERS, DVM
Diplomate, American College of Veterinary Internal Medicine; Diplomate, American College of Veterinary Emergency and Critical Care; Professor Emeritus, Cornell University, Ithaca, New York, USA

AUTHORS

EMILY A. BARRELL, DVM, MSc
Diplomate, American College of Veterinary Internal Medicine; Assistant Professor, Department of Veterinary Population Medicine, University of Minnesota College of Veterinary Medicine, Saint Paul, Minnesota, USA

MARTA CERCONE, DVM, PhD
Diplomate, American College of Veterinary Internal Medicine - Large Animal; Senior Research Associate, Department of Clinical Sciences, Cornell University, Ithaca, New York, USA

MICHELLE DELCO, DVM, PhD
Diplomate, American College of Veterinary Surgeons; Assistant Research Professor, Department of Clinical Sciences, College of Veterinary Medicine, Ithaca, New York, USA

BARBARA DELVESCOVO, DVM, MRCVS, ACVIM
Clinical Instructor, Large Animal Medicine, Cornell University, Ithaca, New York, USA

SALLYANNE L. DENOTTA, DVM, PhD
Diplomate, American College of Veterinary Internal Medicine; Department of Large Animal Clinical Sciences, College of Veterinary Medicine, University of Florida, Gainesville, Florida, USA

THOMAS J. DIVERS, DVM
Diplomate, American College of Veterinary Internal Medicine; Diplomate, American College of Veterinary Emergency and Critical Care; Professor Emeritus, Cornell University, Ithaca, New York, USA

SUSAN L. FUBINI, DVM
Diplomate, American College of Veterinary Surgeons; Professor Large Animal Surgery, Associate Dean for Academic Affairs, Cornell University, Ithaca, New York, USA

TIM MAIR, BVSc, PhD, FRCVS
Diploma in Equine Internal Medicine; Diploma in Equine Soft Tissue Surgery; Diplomate, European College of Equine Internal Medicine; Associate of the European College of Veterinary Diagnostic Imaging; Bell Equine Veterinary Clinic, CVS Ltd, Mereworth, United Kingdom

KATHLEEN R. MULLEN, DVM, MS
Diplomate, American College of Veterinary Internal Medicine - Large Animal Internal Medicine; Associate, Internal Medicine, Littleton Equine Medical Center, Littleton, Colorado, USA

EMIL OLSEN, DVM, PhD
Diplomate, American College of Veterinary Internal Medicine; Diplomate, European College of Equine Internal Medicine; Neurologist and Equine Internist, Veterinary Teaching Hospital (Universitetsdjursjukhuset, UDS), Swedish Veterinary Agricultural University (SLU), Uppsala, Sweden

GABY VAN GALEN, DVM, PhD
Diplomate, European College of Equine Internal Medicine; Diplomate, European College of Veterinary Emergency and Critical Care; Honorary A/Prof Equine Internal Medicine, University of Sydney, Sydney, Australia

Contents

Regulation of renal blood flow is by both extrinsic and intrinsic systems. Intrinsic regulation occurs via the afferent and efferent arterioles and tubuloglomerular feedback mechanisms following activation of the juxtaglomerular apparatus. Mechanisms of acute kidney injury in horses are frequently associated with changes in renal blood flow. Acute tubular necrosis and apoptosis are common in horses following ischemic or toxic insults and in sepsis-associated acute kidney injury. Sepsis-associated renal injury often has a complex mechanism of disease involving both functional and obstructive changes in intrarenal circulation. Acute interstitial nephritis may occur following Leptospira sp infection or can be secondary to tubular necrosis.

Nephrotoxic and hemodynamically mediated disorders are the most common causes of acute renal failure (ARF) in horses and foals. *Leptospira spp.* is the most common infectious cause of ARF. Initial treatments for ARF include elimination of nephrotoxic drugs, correction of predisposing disorders, and fluid therapy to promote diuresis. Horses and foals with polyuric ARF often have a good prognosis, while those with oliguric or anuric ARF have a guarded to poor prognosis. When fluid therapy is unsuccessful in improving urine production, various drug treatments have been used in an attempt to increase urine production, but none are consistently effective in converting oliguria to polyuria.

Chronic kidney disease (CKD) is rare in horses with an overall prevalence reported to be 0.12%. There is often a continuum from Acute Kidney Injury (AKI) to CKD, and patients with CKD may be predisposed to episodes of AKI. The most common clinical signs are non-specific with weight loss, polyuria/polydipsia and ventral edema. Less common clinical signs are poor appetite and performance, dull hair coat, oral ulcerations, gastrointestinal ulceration, gingivitis, dental tartar and diarrhea. Rarely, horses may develop forebrain signs. Creatinine increases when at least 2/3 of kidney function have been lost and a more accurate assessment of kidney function is an estimated glomerular filtration rate measuring iohexol clearance time combined with protein content in the urine. Tubulointerstitial disease and glomerulonephritis are common causes of chronic kidney disease together with pyelonephritis and nephrolithiasis. Dietary changes and avoiding nephrotoxic drugs are key in slowing down the degenerative process.

Urinary disease in the neonatal period can occur with primary congenital renal defects or as a secondary consequence of birth trauma, ischemic injury, nephrotoxic medications, or systemic illness. This article reviews the clinical evaluation of the urinary system in foals and highlights diagnostic and therapeutic features of the most commonly encountered urinary disorders of the equine neonatal patient.

This article describes the most common causes of urine discoloration. The review includes a description of the most common disorders causing hematuria, highlighting clinical presentation, treatments, and pathophysiology. Causes of hemoglobinuria and myoglobinuria together with their mechanisms of renal injury are also reviewed.

Urinary incontinence results from disorders of the lower urinary tract or neurologic diseases either of the nerve supply to the bladder/urethra or within the central nervous system. Congenital causes include patent urachus and ectopic ureter. Coordination of lower urinary tract function involves the interaction of both the sympathetic and parasympathetic system as well as somatic branches of the central nervous system. Well-recognized causes of incontinence include equine herpes virus 1 myeloencephalopathy, polyneuritis equi (neuritis of the cauda equina), and sacral/coccygeal trauma. Idiopathic bladder paralysis is characterized by bladder paralysis and sabulous cystitis in the absence of overt neurologic deficits.

Polyuria and polydipsia are rare, but significant, manifestations of several different diseases of horses. Causes can be endocrine, iatrogenic, psychogenic, infectious, or toxic in nature and can also be due to primary renal disease or diseases of other organs, such as the liver. Although numerous causes of polyuria and polydipsia in horses exist, the most common conditions include chronic kidney disease, pituitary pars intermedia dysfunction, and psychogenic polydipsia with secondary polyuria. Additional testing is dictated by history, other clinical signs, and the results of blood work and/or urinalysis. Prognosis for horses with polyuria and/or polydipsia varies significantly based on the underlying cause.

This article overviews several metabolic disorders associated with renal disease in horses. Included is a discussion of the pathophysiology, clinical signs, and treatment of hyperchloremic metabolic acidosis associated with renal tubular acidosis. Conditions affecting the central nervous system including uremic encephalopathy and hyponatremic encephalopathy secondary to renal disease are presented. Finally, a discussion of the unique features of calcium and phosphorus homeostasis in horses is provided with special emphasis on a recently described syndrome of calcinosis and calciphylaxis of unknown etiology.

Video content accompanies this article at http://www.vetequine. theclinics.com

This article provides a comprehensive review of imaging techniques used to evaluate the equine urinary tract. This overview includes officially recognized modalities and new applications reported in the most current literature. Technical aspects and indications for use of endoscopy and ultrasonography are highlighted. Normal endoscopic and ultrasonographic appearance of the upper and lower urinary tract is described, with characterization of common abnormalities found in patients with hematuria, stranguria, and renal failure. Visual examples of several pathologic conditions from clinical cases are provided. An outline of the main features, potentials, and limitations of radiography, nuclear scintigraphy, and computed tomography is provided.

Urinary surgery in the horse may be challenging. More straightforward procedures, such as urinary bladder or urachal defects, do not usually require specialized equipment or imaging, although laboratory work is helpful. Congenital or acquired conditions of the ureters or kidneys may necessitate advanced diagnostic work-ups including advanced imaging and/or minimally invasive procedures. Some surgery of the lower urinary tract is done in the sedated, standing adult horse. Surgery involving the kidney typically requires general anesthesia. Laparoscopy and associated tools are frequently used. Although many of the surgical procedures discussed are quite involved, they are becoming more commonplace.

VETERINARY CLINICS OF
NORTH AMERICA: EQUINE PRACTICE

SERIES OF RELATED INTEREST

Veterinary Clinics of North America: Food Animal Practice
https://www.vetfood.theclinics.com/

THE CLINICS ARE NOW AVAILABLE ONLINE!
Access your subscription at:
www.theclinics.com

Preface

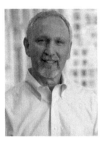

Thomas J. Divers, DVM
Editor

It is a great honor and wonderful opportunity to be guest editor for this *Veterinary Clinics of North America: Equine Practice* issue on Equine Urinary Tract Diseases. The urinary system was my initial organ system of special interest when I began my professional career 47 years ago, so I was excited to edit this issue. I am indebted to Drs. Robert Whitlock and Wayne Crowell at the University of Georgia for stimulating my interest in urinary tract diseases. As time passed, my focus moved to the study of other organ systems in horses, but I never lost that initial interest. Any contributions I have made to the science and clinical practice related to equine urinary tract diseases are very modest compared with others, such as Dr. Hal Schott at Michigan State University and Dr. Warwick Bayly at Washington State University. A quick glimpse at the author references throughout this issue provides an overview of the many contributions those two individuals have made to the field. The last issue of the *Veterinary Clinics of North America: Equine Practice* that focused of Urinary Tract Disorders, edited by Dr. Schott, was 15 years ago, and many advances in the diagnosis and treatments of urinary tract disorders have occurred since that issue. The purpose of the current issue is to provide the most up-to-date information on equine urinary tract disorders focusing on information that is directly applicable to clinical practice. This issue would not have been possible without the excellent chapter contributions from colleagues and close friends, to whom I am gratefully indebted. I would also like to thank others who helped review and prepare the articles, including Susan Branch, Sarah Van Orman, Alexandra Attenasio, and Dr. Nita Irby, my wife and best friend. I also wish to thank Katerina Heidhausen, *Veterinary Clinics of North America: Equine Practice* editor, and Ann Gielou Posedio, developmental editor, and the Elsevier staff for editing this issue. I have had the great pleasure of serving for 5 years as consulting editor for *Veterinary Clinics of North America: Equine Practice* and have thoroughly enjoyed working with both Katerina Heidhausen and Colleen Dietzler (former *Veterinary Clinics of North America: Equine Practice* editor) during that time. I would like to take this opportunity to thank the 24 guest editors and hundreds of article authors who during my time as consulting editor, organized, wrote, and edited outstanding issues on a wide

Vet Clin Equine 38 (2022) ix–x
https://doi.org/10.1016/j.cveq.2022.01.001
0749-0739/22/© 2022 Published by Elsevier Inc.

variety of topics in equine medicine, surgery, and reproduction. I hope the previous issues and this current issue have met the main purpose *of Veterinary Clinics of North America: Equine Practice*: to improve both the standards of care in equine practice and the health of our horses.

Lastly, in my retirement as consultingeEditor, I would like to congratulate the next consulting editor for *Veterinary Clinics of North America: Equine Practice*. I am sure that the *Veterinary Clinics of North America: Equine Practice* will continue to provide outstanding and useful information for practicing equine veterinarians.

Thomas J. Divers, DVM
Cornell University
Ithaca, NY 14853, USA

E-mail address:
Tjd8@cornell.edu

Relevant Equine Renal Anatomy, Physiology, and Mechanisms of Acute Kidney Injury: A Review

Thomas J. Divers, DVM

KEYWORDS

- Equine • Kidney injury • Circulation • Physiology • Mechanisms of disease

KEY FINDINGS

- The equine kidney has some unique anatomic features, such as 2 large collecting ducts (terminal recesses) that drain urine from each pole of the kidney and a short renal crest carrying urine from centrally located papillae into the renal pelvis. This area is predisposed to ischemic necrosis following administration of nonsteroidal antiinflammatory drugs.
- Autoregulation of glomerular blood flow and pressure can occur by direct myogenic responses in the afferent arteriole or via the tubuloglomerular feedback system.
- Ischemic and toxic causes of acute kidney injury predominantly cause acute tubular necrosis and apoptosis.
- Sepsis-associated acute kidney injury often has a complex pathophysiology involving microcirculation dysfunction, inflammation, and coagulopathy with thrombi or fibrin strands in renal vessels.

INTRODUCTION

The pathophysiology of acute kidney injury (AKI) is complex, as is renal circulation and glomerular filtration. The intent of this article is to review the complexity of renal circulation and its effect on glomerular filtration as a prelude to a discussion of mechanisms of AKI and renal failure, with a goal of introducing knowledge that will be helpful in diagnosing, treating, and preventing AKI and failure in horses.

EQUINE RENAL ANATOMY

The equine kidneys are located in the retroperitoneal space of the dorsal abdomen. The combined weight of both kidneys equals approximately 0.3% of body weight.[1]

College of Veterinary Medicine, Cornell University, 930 Campus Road, Ithaca, NY 14853-6401, USA
E-mail address: tjd8@cornell.edu

Vet Clin Equine 38 (2022) 1–12
https://doi.org/10.1016/j.cveq.2021.11.001
0749-0739/22/© 2021 Elsevier Inc. All rights reserved.

The 2 kidneys are usually of similar weight, but this can vary.[1] The renal capsular surfaces are smooth, and the capsule is tightly fitted to the underlying parenchyma. Internal lobations are not present in the adult horse kidney but foal kidneys may exhibit some lobations.[2] On cut section, there is a recognizable division between the renal cortex and medulla, with the cortex appearing brown-red color and granular (caused by the glomeruli). The cortex comprises slightly more than 50% of the kidney volume.[3] The cortex contains approximately 1.0×10^6 nephrons, which are the functional unit of the kidney.[4] Cortical nephrons are nephrons located more superficially in the cortex; they have short tubular loops that U-turn shortly after entering the medulla. Juxtamedullary nephrons are the glomeruli located deep in the cortex near the corticomedullary junction, and their tubules extend deep into the medulla (**Fig. 1**). Cortical nephrons comprise approximately 75% of the nephrons in humans and are the primary nephrons for filtration of plasma, whereas the juxtaglomerular nephrons are most important for concentrating or diluting urine.[5]

The renal medulla comprises approximately 45% of the kidney volume and has a wide inner pale area and a narrower outer red zone.[2,3] The medulla consists primarily of tubules and ducts, surrounded by interstitium, that drain urine toward the renal pelvis. The papillary ducts from each pole of the kidney drain into 1 of 2 long terminal recesses and then into the renal pelvis near the renal crest, whereas papillary ducts located centrally in the medulla open along the approximately 3 cm long renal crest that drains directly into the renal pelvis.[6] A considerable amount of fat is located in each renal pelvis, along with mucous-producing glands whose mucus causes normal equine urine to often seem thick and cloudy.[2] Urine leaves the renal pelvis and kidney via the proximal ureter, which is located at the renal hilus, along with the renal arteries and vein.

RENAL BLOOD FLOW

Blood flow to the kidney normally comprises approximately 20% to 25% of total cardiac output in humans, and in the horse it has been measured to be 22%.[7,8] This relatively high blood flow is required to meet the extensive glomerular filtration process and the metabolic needs of the relatively underperfused renal medulla.[8] The renal cortex receives more than 90% of the total renal blood flow and has a low oxygen extraction.[9] The medulla, despite having a high metabolic rate associated with the active resorption and secretion of ions there, receives less than 10% of the renal blood flow and has a high oxygen extraction.[5,8] Blood enters the renal cortex via the renal artery and its divisions at the hilus; some horses also have an accessory artery that enters the cortex on the medial aspect of the kidney.[10] Blood flows from the main renal arteries through the interlobar arteries to the arcuate arteries that run between the cortex and medulla. The arcuate arteries give rise to cortical interlobular arteries (also called cortical radial arteries) that ascend toward the renal capsule. These arteries are end arteries and are susceptible to focal ischemic necrosis.[11] Branches from the cortical interlobular arteries give rise to the very important afferent arterioles that individually supply blood to the capillary bed of each glomerulus. After flowing through the glomerular capillary bed, blood leaves each glomerulus via an efferent arteriole. This precisely arranged 2-arteriole system at the glomerulus is a circulatory pattern unique to the kidney, as is the high-pressure capillary bed in the glomerulus. Afferent and efferent arterioles are critically important for maintaining an appropriate glomerular perfusion pressure and filtration rate (GFR). Next, most of the blood from the efferent arterioles flows through capillaries called peritubular capillaries, which run in close proximity to the cortical tubules before leaving the kidney via a set of venous

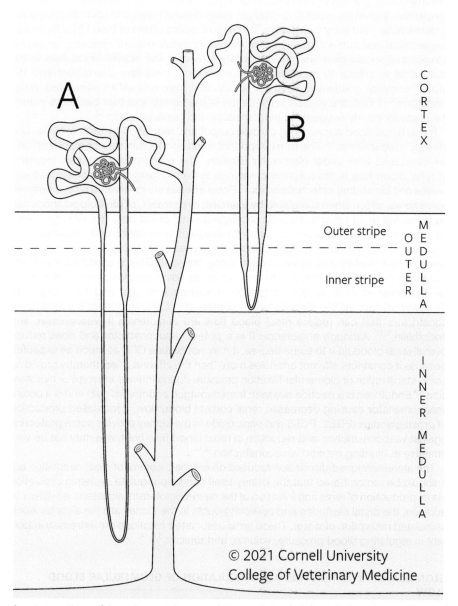

A

B

CORTEX

Outer stripe

Inner stripe

OUTER

MEDULLA

INNER MEDULLA

Fig. 1. Location of long-looped juxtamedullary nephron (A) and short-looped cortical nephron (B) in the kidney. Image used with permission of Cornell University College of Veterinary Medicine.

branches and ultimately into the renal vein that exits the kidney at the hilus near the renal arteries and proximal ureter. Efferent arterioles from juxtamedullary glomeruli nephrons flow into the medulla as physiologically unique parallel bundles of vessels called *vasa recta*.[12,13] The outer most vessels in the *vasa recta* bundle give rise to "slow flow" capillaries that surround each loop of Henle and collecting duct of the juxtamedullary glomeruli nephrons. *Vasa recta* vessels are part of the *countercurrent mechanism* important in solute exchange, water reabsorption, and maintenance of the hyperosmotic medullary interstitium.[12] The *vasa recta* pattern of blood flow facilitates oxygenation and nutrient supply to the medullary tissue without removing excessive solutes that would decrease the medullary tonicity.[8] The slower blood flow in the *vasa recta* is critical to maintaining the hypertonic medullary interstitium and the proper osmolar gradient needed for antidiuretic hormone (ADH)-stimulated water resorption.[5,12] Only the vessels in the center of the bundle and their capillaries supply the *relatively* poorly oxygenated inner medulla and papilla/crest.[12,13]

Renal blood flood depends on cardiac output and regulation by both extrinsic and intrinsic mechanisms.[14] The most important intrinsic mechanisms of autoregulation are discussed later under glomerular filtration. The predominant extrinsic regulator of renal blood flow is the autonomic nervous system, mostly by way of sympathetic nerves and circulating catecholamines.[15] Renal arteries are innervated by sympathetic nerve fibers, which when stimulated by exercise, excitement, or physiologic shock can constrict the renal vessels, thereby decreasing renal blood flow and GFR.[8,15] Renal vasoconstriction can also occur following release of epinephrine and norepinephrine from the adrenal medulla during excitement.[5] Horses undergoing high-intensity exercise showed marked decreases in renal blood flow and GFR in association with the increased sympathetic activity.[7] In another study using treadmill exercised horses, GFR decreased 40% to 50% with only moderate exercise, and GFR began to decrease as soon as the horses started exercising.[16] Other important humoral vasoconstrictors that can reduce renal blood flow are angiotensin II, vasopressin, and endothelin.[5,17] Although angiotensin II is a potent vasoconstrictor and does reduce overall renal blood flow to some degree, it may not reduce GFR as much as expected because it constricts efferent arterioles more than the afferent ones, thereby providing some stabilization of glomerular filtration pressure during intense exercise or hypotension.[18] Endothelin is a peptide released from damaged endothelial cells and is a potent vasoconstrictor causing decreased renal cortical blood flow.[19] Increased production of prostaglandins (PGE2, PGI2) and nitric oxide in the kidney provide some protection against vasoconstriction and reduction in renal blood flow but these may not be very effective at blunting marked vasoconstriction.[8,14]

The aforementioned discussion focused on extrinsic control of renal circulation but it should be remembered that the kidney itself can help regulate systemic circulation via its production of renin and initiation of the renin-angiotensin-aldosterone system. In addition, the distal nephrons and collecting ducts in the kidney are the sites for ADH-stimulated resorption of water. These renal associated functions are extremely important in regulating blood pressure, volume, and tonicity.[5,8,14]

GLOMERULAR FILTRATION AND AUTOREGULATION OF GLOMERULAR BLOOD FLOW

The functional unit of the kidney is the nephron, composed of a glomerulus and a network of tubes distally. Each glomerulus is surrounded by a Bowman capsule, which has a space (Bowman space) that collects the glomerular filtrate, which then drains into the proximal renal tubule.[5,14] Although not the only function, the primary function of the nephron is to filter blood and regulate both plasma ion concentrations and fluid balance.[20]

GFR is determined by (1) blood flow to the glomerulus; (2) perfusion pressure at the glomerulus; (3) surface area of the glomerular capillaries; (4) efficiency of the glomerular capillary membrane; and (5) the hydrostatic and oncotic pressure differences between the glomerular capillaries and Bowman space.[12] Normally, approximately 20% of the renal plasma flow is filtered across the glomerular membrane (filtration fraction).[12] The health of the glomerular filtration barrier, renal blood flow, and glomerular perfusion pressures are the most important determinants of GFR.[11,12] Oncotic pressure differences between Bowman space and the glomerular capillaries or increased hydrostatic pressure in Bowman space also affect GFR. These are usually minor compared with the effect of renal blood flow and glomerular hydrostatic pressure on GFR.[11] Tubular obstruction, complete or partial, increases hydrostatic pressure in Bowman space and may significantly inhibit GFR.[11]

An important and unique intrarenal mechanism for regulating GFR is the glomerular 2-artery system: afferent and efferent arterioles that respectively supply blood to and drain blood from the glomerular capillary bed. Autoregulation of pressure in these 2 arterioles occurs in an attempt to maintain perfusion pressures and GFR when challenged by changes in systemic blood pressure (hypotension or hypertension) or renal blood flow.[5,12,21]

Autoregulation of glomerular arteriole pressures occurs predominantly in the afferent and efferent arterioles by 2 mechanisms, a direct myogenic response to pressure changes and the tubuloglomerular feedback system.[11,12] *Myogenic responses* in the muscular wall of the afferent and efferent arterioles occur almost immediately following renal artery pressure changes.[11] For example, during systemic hypotension renal afferent arteriolar smooth muscle relaxes, lowering resistance in an effort to maintain renal blood flow and GFR. The opposite occurs during hypertension to protect the glomerular membranes.[5,11,12,14] Normally, pressure in the afferent arteriole entering the glomerulus and in the efferent arteriole leaving the glomerulus are very similar (note that pressure in the efferent arteriole declines rapidly after leaving the glomerulus in order to supply the low-pressure, slower flow peritubular capillaries).[12] If the afferent and efferent arterioles respond identically to a situation, there is minimal effect on GFR. On the other hand, if they respond differently, GFR is altered. For example, angiotensin II is known to constrict the efferent arteriole more than the afferent arteriole, and during hypotensive episodes this helps maintain glomerular capillary pressure and GFR.[5,8] In summary, pressure changes in the afferent and efferent arteriole allow the kidney to regulate GFR independent of renal blood flow.[12,15,21] The changes in pressure between the 2 arteries is likely unpredictable in patients who are hemodynamically unstable, such as during sepsis, hemorrhage, and so on,[22] making it difficult to select vasopressor therapy when treating a horse with oliguria and increasing azotemia.

Tubuloglomerular (TG) feedback mechanisms are a second important means of autoregulation of renal blood flow and GFR.[5,8,11,14] The most important anatomic component of the TG feedback mechanism involved in autoregulation of renal blood flow is the juxtaglomerular apparatus (JGA).[5,12] The JGA is found in each nephron at the confluence of the afferent arteriole, efferent arteriole, and the distal convoluted tubule. The JGA is composed of granular cells (also called juxtaglomerular cells and located in the walls of afferent arterioles), extraglomerular mesangial cells (located just outside of Bowman capsule between the afferent and efferent arterioles), and macula densa cells (specialized cells within the wall of the distal convoluted tubule) (**Fig. 2**). The macula densa cells sense changes in sodium chloride concentrations and flow rate of the filtrate.[5,14] As GFR decreases (eg, during hypotension) there is a decrease in tubular flow rate, allowing more time for sodium and chloride reabsorption in the proximal tubules, resulting in low sodium and chloride concentrations reaching the macula densa cells. When this occurs, the macula densa cells increase their release of nitric oxide and vasodilatory prostaglandins, causing their adjacent

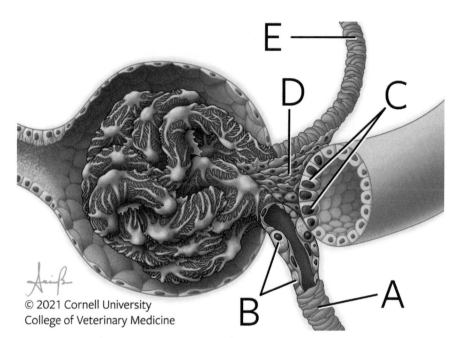

Fig. 2. Anatomy of the juxtaglomerular apparatus (JGA). (A) Afferent arteriole, (B) granular cells, (C) macula densa cells in the wall of the distal tubule, (D) mesangial cells, and (E) efferent arteriole. Bowman capsule and glomerular capillaries are to the left. Image used with permission of Cornell University College of Veterinary Medicine.

afferent arteriole to dilate and increase blood flow in an effort to stabilize GFR in that nephron. Simultaneously, renin is secreted from the granular cells, activating the renin-angiotensin system and preferentially constricting the efferent arteriole to increase glomerular perfusion pressure and help maintain GFR.[23] The opposite occurs following an increase in GFR causing high salt concentration and high tubular flow at the site of macula densa cells that then release ATP and its metabolite adenosine causing the afferent arteriole to constrict, decreasing blood flow to the glomerulus. The autoregulation of renal hemodynamics and GFR discussed earlier are usually excellent at maintaining GFR when changes in blood pressure are modest but with severe changes in blood pressure, in either direction, the success of autoregulation in maintaining GFR is diminished.[21]

TG mechanisms not only help regulate glomerular pressures and GFR but also have significant effects on systemic blood pressure via activation of the renin-angiotensin system. Angiotensin II is also the primary factor controlling the release of aldosterone from the adrenal gland.[5] Increases in serum aldosterone will increase sodium resorption from the distal tubules and collecting ducts that can increase intravascular volume within hours.

MECHANISMS OF ACUTE KIDNEY INJURY

AKI is a term used to describe early and often nonclinical renal injury. AKI is defined by one or more of the following: (1) increased serum creatinine of 0.3 mg/dL or greater within 48 hours, (2) increased serum creatinine 1.5 times baseline or more within 7 days, or (3) oliguria of 6 hours duration in the face of adequate hydration status.[23] The term AKI has clinical implications when evaluated over time and with clinical judgment but without this information it may not tell us much about the degree of kidney injury or function.[23] In addition, oliguria may not be readily detected in horses with AKI due to difficulty in quantitating urine production. AKI was a relatively common equine disorder in one study where 14.8% of hospitalized horses developed AKI.[24] In most cases, AKI will not progress to acute renal failure (ARF) if proper treatment is provided. ARF occurs following the loss of approximately 75% or greater nephron function and reduced ability to excrete waste products and maintain fluid and electrolyte homeostasis.[20] When ARF occurs in horses, the mortality rate can be high depending upon the cause and promptness of treatment.[25,26]

AKI and ARF may occur from prerenal, intrarenal, or postrenal causes, with each having different, but often overlapping, pathophysiology. Although the precise pathophysiologic mechanisms of AKI and ARF in horses are not well documented, we can make assumptions regarding possible mechanisms based on studies in other species.[11,20]

Prerenal mechanisms causing AKI in horses are a result of decreased blood flow to the kidneys in association with dehydration and/or hypotension. A decrease in blood flow and increase in serum protein concentration secondary to dehydration decreases glomerular capillary hydrostatic pressure and increases capillary oncotic pressure, respectively, with both causing a decrease in GFR, but due to the protective autoregulation of renal blood flow functional changes in GFR may not occur unless there is a 25% or greater reduction in blood flow.[8,11,14] If the decrease in renal blood flow persists and/or nonsteroidal antiinflammatory drugs (NSAIDs) are administered, tubular injury may occur.

TUBULAR ISCHEMIA

Tubular epithelial cells (TECs) are predisposed to ischemic injury due to their high surface area needed for reabsorption and active transport systems and their high metabolism rate and oxygen demand.[27] If a circulating blood volume deficit or hypotension is sufficiently severe, TECs may not receive adequate oxygen and nutrients from adjacent peritubular capillaries leading to tubular necrosis, apoptosis, and dysfunction.[11,13] Preferential constriction of the efferent arteriole by angiotensin II, in an attempt to maintain glomerular perfusion pressure and GFR, can further decrease peritubular capillary flow. Some nephron segments seem to be more susceptible to the relative hypoxia and are unable to shift to anaerobic metabolism under low oxygen conditions.[13] This may be especially true of the proximal tubules and the ascending loop of Henle, both of which are active transport sites for electrolyte absorption and sites of high metabolic activity.[13,27] In addition, both of these nephron segments dip into the outer medulla, which has less oxygen than the cortex and is a known site for capillary congestion, potentiating additional ischemic injury to nephrons in this area.[9] The tubular injury associated with ischemia can be seen as patchy areas of necrosis but this may not always be obvious on microscopic examination.[27] Effacement and loss of proximal tubule brush border, patchy loss of tubule cells, focal areas of proximal tubular dilation, and tubular casts may also be noted.[20,28] TEC injury can lead to tubular contents leaking into the nearby interstitium causing interstitial edema.[11,20] Individual nephrons can become partially or even completely obstructed from sloughing epithelial casts and from interstitial edema compressing the tubule, both of which cause increased intraluminal tubular pressure.[11] The increased intraluminal pressure will increase pressure in Bowman space and decrease individual nephron's GFR. Blood from obstructed or dysfunctional nephrons may be redirected to nephrons that are more functional.

TOXIC TUBULAR NECROSIS AND APOPTOSIS

Toxic tubular necrosis in horses most commonly occurs when aminoglycoside or tetra-cycline antibiotics are administered to dehydrated or hypotensive animals[29]; this may also occur following prolonged drug administration. High concentrations of a nephro-toxic drug or chemical in the glomerular filtrate during decreased urine flow, as might occur with dehydration, can result in increased absorption of the drug into the TEC. TEC damage may be from direct toxic effects of drugs or their metabolites.[20,30] The mechanism of TEC damage can vary between drugs but free radical formation, exces-sive intracellular calcium, mitochondrial injury, and decreased ATP are some common mechanisms of cell injury.[11,20,27,30,31] Mechanisms of TEC injury from aminoglycosides are described and include loss of protein synthesis, reduction of the mitochondrial func-tion, and consequent cell death.[30] Microscopic findings in the kidney with toxic ne-phropathy include flattening of TECs and detachment and shedding of tubular cells and protein into the tubule lumens forming obstructing casts, similar to what is seen with ischemic tubular necrosis.[11,20] Obstruction of tubular lumens causes an increase in Bowman capsule pressure, decreasing that individual nephron's GFR.

Both ischemic and nephrotoxic ARF often have a good prognosis if the horse is not oliguric and if the degree of damage to the tubular basement membrane is modest. Damage to the basement membrane may be more common with ischemic tubular ne-crosis although severe damage can occur from nephrotoxic drugs. Morphologic re-covery of the kidney may occur within 2 to 3 weeks following resolution of an ischemic or toxic insult.[20] Some horses may have complete clinical recovery from ischemic or nephrotoxic AKI with serum creatinine or other markers of GRF returning to normal range but others may recover clinically yet maintain some elevation in serum creatinine associated with permanent loss of a significant number of nephrons in spite of hypertrophy of other nephrons.[20] Patients with persistent oliguria or anuria are un-likely to recover. An important clinical observation is that with both aminoglycoside and tetracycline nephrotoxicity, serum creatinine often continues to increase for 2 to 3 days after discontinuing the nephrotoxic drug and beginning fluid therapy; this is likely due in part to residual drug in circulation and high residues in the kidney.

NONSTEROIDAL ANTIINFLAMMATORY DRUG NEPHROTOXICITY

NSAID nephrotoxicity is a common cause of AKI in horses, but fulminant ARF following NSAID toxicity is uncommon.[29] Prostaglandins with their vasodilatation effect are help-ful in maintaining GFR and preserving renal blood flow, especially in fluid-depleted state. Localized PG synthesis (PGI_2, PGE_2, PGD_2) causes vasodilatation of afferent arteriole and increases renal perfusion.[32] PGI_2 and PGE_2 are especially important in protecting the relatively blood-deprived medulla against hypoperfusion and hypoxia.[14,27,33] Blood flow to this normally poorly oxygenated region of the kidney is via the slow-flowing *vasa recta* capillaries.[8] The predominant renal lesion in the horse following NSAID administra-tion is focal coagulative ischemic necrosis of the renal crest and the corresponding inner medulla.[33] Secondary tubular necrosis, interstitial inflammation, and atrophy of the cor-responding glomerular tufts may also occur.[33] Dehydration and intense athletic activity are risk factors for NSAID-induced renal disease.[33] Adult horses are most commonly affected, and most of the affected horses have bilateral disease.[33]

HEMODYNAMICALLY MEDIATED OR SEPSIS-ASSOCIATED NEPHROPATHY

Hemodynamically mediated (also sometimes referred to as vasomotor or sepsis associated) nephropathy is a documented cause of ARF in horses and foals that have sepsis or systemic inflammatory disease.[26,34,35] Sepsis-associated AKI is common in humans, and the pathophysiology is believed to be associated with microcirculation dysfunction, inflammation, coagulopathy, and possibly metabolic reprogramming of the TECs in response to sepsis.[22,36] Although some of these proposed mechanisms of disease remain unproved, there is general agreement that the pathophysiology is more complex than the pathophysiology of toxic and ischemic tubular necrosis.[36] In horses, there is often evidence of enhanced coagulation and disseminated intravascular coagulation (**Fig. 3**).[26,34,35,37] In a neonatal foal sepsis study, fibrin deposition in the microcirculation of the kidneys of nonsurviving foals was common in 14 of 32 nonsurviving foals, some of which had ARF.[34] Renal cortical necrosis with hemorrhage occurred in 5 of the 32 nonsurviving foals. Activation of the coagulation cascade in response to inflammatory mediators and cellular injury can cause vascular thrombosis in the equine kidney.[26] Decreases in renal blood flow resulting from hypotension or systemic inflammatory disease are likely part of the mechanism of disease, as is dysregulation of the pressure balance between the afferent and efferent arterioles.[22,36] With severe decreases in renal blood flow, outer cortical nephrons can be most severely affected.[20] Regardless of the mechanisms, hemodynamic or sepsis-mediated ARF is a very complex disorder making therapeutic choices challenging.[13,22] With hemodynamically mediated ARF, affected horses may suffer a rapid and progressive azotemia, which can progress quickly to uremia and then death, especially in horses that are oliguric or anuric.[26]

PIGMENT NEPHROPATHY

ARF in association with either myoglobinuria or hemoglobinuria is likely a combination of vasomotor and nephrotoxic mechanisms of disease. With either myopathy/myositis or hemolytic anemia, pronounced sympathetic stimulation may occur with release of catecholamines that can negatively affect renal blood flow. These disorders can also increase coagulation and systemic inflammatory responses, further affecting renal hemodynamics.[38] Hemolysis or a decrease in total red blood cells from any cause can also increase the likelihood of developing tubular hypoxia. Although myoglobin and hemoglobin may only have modest direct toxic effects on the tubular epithelium of healthy animals, these pigments can cause cytotoxicity and oxidative tubular epithelial damage and obstruct tubular casts that may form especially in dehydrated or hypotensive horses.[39,40]

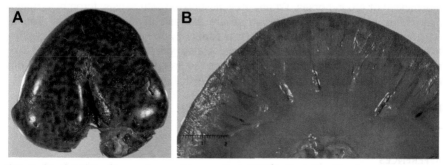

Figs. 3. (*A, B*) Kidney from a 4-year-old mare that died from peritonitis, disseminated intravascular coagulation, and acute, anuric renal failure. Hemorrhages and necrosis were present symmetrically throughout both renal cortices.

ACUTE INTERSTITIAL NEPHRITIS

Acute interstitial nephritis as a primary mechanism of ARF in horses is uncommon but may occur during acute *Leptospira* sp infection or from immune reactions. Leptospirosis causes AKI and ARF because of the organism's renal trophism that occurs following or concurrent with bacteremia.[41,42] The injury to the kidney is believed to be due to both a direct injury caused by the organism and secondary to the immune inflammatory response. Lipopolysaccharide and other outer membrane proteins activate the immune response.[43] The outer protein surface antigen, LipL32 found in all pathogenic leptospiral organisms, can also damage both the renal interstitium and TECs by activating proinflammatory proteins.[44] The renal lesions can include acute tubular necrosis and tubulointerstitial nephritis characterized by interstitial edema and dense local infiltrates of neutrophils and mononuclear cells.[20,41]

OBSTRUCTIVE NEPHROPATHY

Obstructive nephropathy, an infrequent cause of ARF in horses, may occur following acute urethral obstruction or obstruction to both ureters that is sometimes seen in neonatal foals (personal communication). One of the earliest physiologic events following obstruction to urine flow is a retrograde increase in hydrostatic pressure in the renal tubules and Bowman space.[45] This increase in pressure outside of the glomerulus, combined with glomerular mesangial cell contraction, has a negative effect on glomerular filtration. After an initial increase in renal blood flow, possibly to offset the early increase in tubular pressure, vasoconstriction of the afferent arteriole occurs leading to decreased glomerular blood flow and further reductions in GFR.[45,46] The pronounced decrease in GFR caused by obstruction to urine flow prevents renal elimination of potassium, and life-threatening hyperkalemia is a common consequence. Obstruction to urine flow and decreased blood flow in the peritubular capillaries have several adverse effects on tubular integrity and function, including causing abnormalities in interstitial salt and water balances and a decrease in medullary tonicity.[46] This decrease in the tonicity of the renal medulla is one mechanism leading to the marked polyuria that often occurs following correction of urinary obstructions. Following prolonged urinary obstruction, the renal pelvis enlarges, renal medullary tissue is lost, and hydronephrosis develops. With prolonged obstruction in only one kidney, that kidney's parenchyma will eventually atrophy due to loss of blood flow, and the intact kidney will hypertrophy.[45,46]

In conclusion, AKI is most common in horses due to ischemic, nephrotoxic, or sepsis-associated mechanisms. Dysfunction of renal circulation is often part of the mechanism of AKI in horses. When AKI is associated with sepsis, thrombi formation may occur in renal vessels causing severe necrosis of the renal cortex. Tubular obstruction due to the presence of casts is especially common in horses with nephrotoxic AKI. Pigment nephropathy is likely associated with both hemodynamic and toxic mechanisms of disease. Obstructive causes, acute severe glomerulonephritis, and acute pyelonephritis are infrequent causes of ARF in horses.

DISCLOSURE

The author has nothing to disclose.

REFERENCES

1. Duncan JT. The weight of the kidneys in the horse. J Comp Pathol Ther 1903;16: 225–57.

2. Singh B. Dyce, Sack, and Wensing's textbook of veterinary anatomy. Philadelphia, Pennsylvania: Elsevier-Saunders; 2017. p. 550–1.
3. Bolat D, Bahar S, Tipirdamaz S, et al. Comparison of the morphometric features of the left and right horse kidneys: a stereological approach. Anat Histol Embryol 2013;42:448–52.
4. Beech DJ, Sibbons PD, Rossdale PD. Organogenesis of lung and kidney in thoroughbreds and ponies. Equine Vet J 2001;33:438–45.
5. Hall JE. Renal glomerular filtration, renal blood flow. In: Hall JE, editor. Guyton and Hall textbook of Medical physiology. 13th edition. Maryland Heights, (MD): Elsevier; 2016. p. 335–47.
6. Pasquel SG, Agnew D, Nelson N, et al. Ureteropyeloscopic anatomy of the renal pelvis of the horse. Equine Vet J 2013;45:31–8.
7. Schott HC, Hodgson DR, Bayly WM, et al. Renal responses to high intensity exercise. In: Gillespie JR, Robinson NE, editors. Equine exercise physiology. Davis, California: ICEEP Publications; 1991. p. 361.
8. Sjaastad OV, Sand O, Hove K. Pathophysiology of domestic animals. 2nd edition. Oslo, Norway: Scandinavian Veterinary Press; 2010. p. 465–79.
9. Ray S, Mason J, O'Connor PM. Ischemic renal injury: can renal anatomy and associated vascular congestion explain why the medulla and not the cortex is where the trouble starts. Semin Nephrol 2019;39:520–9.
10. Pujol R, De Fourmestraux C, Symoens A, et al. Retroperitoneoscopy in the horse: anatomical study of the retroperitoneal perirenal space and description of a surgical approach. Equine Vet J 2021;153:364–72.
11. Breshears MA, Confer AW. The urinary system. In: Pathologic basis of veterinary disease. 6th edition. Maryland Heights, (MD): Elsevier; 2017. p. 617–32.
12. Eaton DS, Pooler JP. Renal blood flow and glomerular filtration, . Vander's renal physiology. 9th edition. New York, (NY): McGraw-Hill Education; 2018. p. 20–35.
13. Scholz H, Bolvin FJ, Schmidt-Ott KM, et al. Kidney physiology and susceptibility to acute kidney injury: implications for renoprotection. Nat Rev Nephrol 2021;17: 335–49.
14. Verlander JW. Renal physiology. In: Klein BG, editor. Cunningham's textbook of veterinary physiology. 5th ed. Philadelphia, (PA): WB Saunders; 2013. p. 460–6.
15. Johns EJ, Kopp UC, DiBona GF. Neural control of renal function. Compr Physiol 2011;1:731–67.
16. Gleadhill A, Marlin D, Harris PA, et al. Reduction of renal function in exercising horses. Equine Vet J 2000;32:509–14.
17. Navar LG, Inscho EW, Majid SA, et al. Paracrine regulation of the renal microcirculation. Physiol Rev 1996;76:425–536.
18. Levens NR, Peach MJ, Carey RM. Role of the intrarenal renin-angiotensin system in the control of renal function. Circ Res 1981;48:157–67.
19. Guan Z, VanBeusecum JP, Inscho EW. Endothelin and the renal microcirculation. Semin Nephrol 2015;35:145–55.
20. Cianciolo R, Mohr FC. The urinary system. In: Maxie MG, editor. Jubb Kennedy and Palmer Pathology of Domestic animals. Maryland Heights, (MD): Elsevier; 2015. p. 376–464.
21. Suarez J, Busse LW. New strategies to optimize renal haemodynamics. Curr Opin Crit Care 2020;26:536–42.
22. Ma S, Evans RG, Iguchi N, et al. Sepsis-induced acute kidney injury: A disease of the microcirculation. Mcrocirculation 2019;26:E12483.
23. Barasch J, Zager R, Bonventre JV. Acute kidney injury: a problem of definition. Lancet 2017;389:779–81.

24. Savage VL, Marr CM, Bailey M, et al. Prevalence of acute kidney injury in a population of hospitalized horses. J Vet Intern Med 2019;33:2294–301.
25. Groover ES, Woolums AR, Cole DJ, et al. Risk factors associated with renal insufficiency in horses with primary gastrointestinal disease: 26 cases (2000–2003). J Am Vet Med Assoc 2006;228:572–7.
26. Divers TJ, Whitlock RH, Byars TD, et al. Acute renal failure in six horses resulting from haemodynamic causes. Equine Vet J 1987;19:178–84.
27. Alpers CE, Chang A. The kidney. In: Kumar V, Abbas AK, Aster JC, editors. Robbins and Cotran pathologic basis of disease. 9th edition. Maryland Heights, MD: Elsevier; 2015. p. 927–30.
28. Devarajan P. Update on mechaisms of ischemic acute kidney disease. J Am Soc Nephrol 2006;17:1503–20.
29. Bartol JM, Divers TJ, Perkins GA. Nephrotoxicant-induced acute renal failure in five horses. Compend Continuing Education Practicing Veterinarian 2000;22:870–6.
30. Perazella MA. Drug-induced acute kidney injury: diverse mechanisms of tubular injury. Curr Opin Crit Care 2019;25:550–7.
31. Barnett LMA, Cummings BS. Nephrotoxicity and renal pathophysiology: a contemporary perspective. Toxicol Sci 2018;164:379–90.
32. Bindu S, Mazumder S, Bandyopadhyay U. Non-steroidal anti-inflammatory drugs (NSAIDs) and organ damage: a current perspective. Biochem Pharmacol 2020;180:114147.
33. Read WK. Renal medullary crest necrosis associated with phenylbutazone therapy in horses. Vet Pathol 1983;20:662–9.
34. Cotovio M, Monreal L, Armengo L, et al. Fibrin deposits and organ failure in newborn foals with severe septicemia. J Vet Intern Med 2008;22:1403–10.
35. Dickinson CE, Gould DH, Davidson AH, et al. Hemolytic-uremic syndrome in a postpartum mare concurrent with encephalopathy in the neonatal foal. J Vet Diagn Invest 2008;20:239–42.
36. Manrique-Caballero CL, Del Rio-Pertuz G, Gomez H. Sepsis-associated acute kidney injury. Crit Care Clin 2021;37:279–301.
37. MacLachlan NJ, Divers TJ. Hemolytic anemia and fibrinoid change of renal vessels in a horse. J Am Vet Med Assoc 1982;181:716–7.
38. Van Avondt K, Nur E, Zeerleder S. Mechanisms of haemolysis-induced kidney injury. Nat Rev Nephrol 2019;15:671–92.
39. Divers TJ, George LW, George JW. Hemolytic anemia in horses after the ingestion of red maple leaves. J Am Vet Med Assoc 1982;180:300–2.
40. el-Ashker MR. Acute kidney injury mediated by oxidative stress in Egyptian horses with exertional rhabdomyolysi. Vet Res Commun 2011;35:35.
41. Frellstedt L, Slovis NM. Acute renal disease from Leptospira interrogans in three yearlings from the same farm. Equine Vet Educ 2009;21:478–84.
42. Divers TJ, Byars TD, Shin SJ. Renal dysfunction associated with infection of Leptospira interrogans in a horse. J Am Vet Med Assoc 1992;201(9):1391–2.
43. da Silva GBJ, Srisawat N, Galdino GS, et al. Acute kidney injury in leptospirosis: overview and perspectives. Asian Pac J Trop Med 2018;11:549–54.
44. Haake DA, Levett PN. Leptospirosis in humans. Curr Top Micriology Immunol 2015;387:65–97.
45. Klahr S, Harris K, Purkerson M. Effects of obstruction on renal functions. Pediatr Nephrol 1988;2:34–42.
46. Klahr PDS. Pathophysiology of obstructive nephropathy. Kidney Int 1983;23:414–26.

Acute Kidney Injury and Renal Failure in Horses

Thomas J. Divers, DVM

KEYWORDS

- Equine • Acute renal failure • Causes • Diagnosis • Treatments • Prevention

KEY POINTS

- Acute renal failure (ARF) is most commonly caused by hemodynamic alterations in renal function secondary to severe systemic illness
- Nephrotoxic drug administration is another common cause of ARF, with dehydration being a risk factor.
- Horses and foals with polyuric ARF are easier to medically manage and have a better prognosis than do horses and foals with oliguric renal failure

INTRODUCTION

Acute kidney injury (AKI) is a common occurrence in hospitalized horses.[1] Fortunately, most equine cases of AKI do not progress to fulminant acute renal failure (ARF). When ARF occurs in horses and foals in either hospital or field practice, it is most commonly associated with hemodynamic or nephrotoxic causes.[2] In human medicine, the term AKI is used when there has been an increase in serum creatinine of 0.3 mg/dL or greater within the past 48 hours. AKI would therefore include both mild and severe changes in renal function. The term ARF often suffers from not having a precise definition, but in the following article ARF is used to describe an advanced decline in glomerular filtration that occurs over hours or days, often resulting in clinical findings directly attributed to the marked decrease in glomerular filtration rate (GFR).[3] The aims of this article are to review causes of ARF in horses and foals and provide guidelines for diagnosis, treatments, and prognosis that might be useful in clinical practice.

CAUSES OF ACUTE RENAL FAILURE

The most frequent causes of ARF in equines are those associated with either hemodynamic or nephrotoxic mechanisms.[2,4] Obstructive nephropathy and interstitial nephritis are infrequent causes of ARF and acute glomerulopathies are rare in horses.

College of Veterinary Medicine, Cornell University, 930 Campus Road, Ithaca, NY 14853-6401, USA
E-mail address: tjd8@cornell.edu

Vet Clin Equine 38 (2022) 13–24
https://doi.org/10.1016/j.cveq.2021.11.002
vetequine.theclinics.com

Horses with hemodynamically mediated ARF, also referred to as vasomotor or sepsis-associated ARF, commonly have a predisposing systemic inflammatory disorder. Hypotension and disseminated intravascular coagulation were frequent findings in adult horses and foals with sepsis-associated ARF.[5,6] Horses with colic may also develop vasomotor nephropathy and AFR. This seems more common when sepsis, hypotension, and abdominal distention persist following surgery. Neonatal foals with respiratory dysfunction or neonatal encephalopathy occasionally develop ARF, but the mechanism is unclear.[7] Acute heart failure and hemorrhage can result in hemodynamically mediated ARF secondary to hypotension and/or hypoxia.[8]

There are several nephrotoxins reported to cause ARF in horses.[2,4] Aminoglycosides and oxytetracycline are the most common antibiotics known to cause ARF,[9] although the incidence of aminoglycoside- induced ARF has seemingly decreased in the last 25 years with the change to once daily dosing. Gentamicin and amikacin are both causes of ARF in horses and foals, but gentamicin is more nephrotoxic than amikacin.[10] Gentamicin, amikacin, and oxytetracycline are most likely to cause renal failure when administered to dehydrated or hypotensive equines.[9] Although uncommon, foals administered a single large dose of oxytetracycline as treatment for contracted tendons have developed ARF.[11] Foals that are unable to stand frequently or long enough to nurse well might be at higher risk of ARF when administered high doses of oxytetracycline. Nonsteroidal anti-inflammatory drug (NSAID) administration is not a common cause of ARF in horses unless hemodynamic risk factors exist. NSAIDs can occasionally cause ARF when administered at high doses to horses with severe laminitis.[9] Although there are no published data, this author has evaluated several horses with ARF associated with bisphosphonate drug administration. This may be more frequent when the bisphosphonate treatment is paired with an NSAID, but I am aware of cases of ARF that occurred following only bisphosphonate treatment. A recent study found that horses frequently have nonclinical increases in serum creatinine following administration of a bisphosphonate drug.[12]

Equine ARF associated with myopathy and hemolysis is relatively common.[13–16] The mechanisms likely include both hemodynamic and nephrotoxic components. The vasomotor component in horses with myopathy could be a result of increased catecholamine activity on renal vasculature or coagulopathy and hypoxia associated with hemolytic disorders. Tubular epithelial damage and cast formation causing tubular obstruction likely play a role in the disease process.

Idiosyncratic or immune-related drug reaction can cause ARF.[17] The author has observed this occasionally in horses in association with intravenous administration of non-nephrotoxic antibiotics, vitamins or hematinics and on rare occasion, following a routine intramuscular administered vaccine. These are likely immune reactions as the horses usually have immediate signs of anaphylaxis that subside before developing signs of uremia 48 to 72 hours later. *Leptospira* spp is the most common infectious cause of ARF.[18,19]

CLINICAL SIGNS

Often the clinical signs of ARF in horses and foals are more the result of the predisposing disease such as diarrhea or septic shock rather than renal failure itself. Some adult horses with acute oliguric renal failure present with colic. The colic signs might be caused by increased pressure within the renal capsule, but this is not proven. Colic signs in horses with ARF include restlessness and frequent pawing. More specific signs directly related to renal failure are those caused by uremia.[2] Renal failure cases associated with a 1-hit insult such as myopathy or an adverse drug reaction often develop clinical signs associated with uremia 3 days later, as it may take 3 days for the uremic toxins to reach levels that affect attitude and appetite. Fever is not a common finding in horses with ARF unless it is associated with a predisposing disease like colitis or bacteremia. When fever is present with ARF, and a predisposing cause is not obvious, leptospirosis should be considered as a possible cause.[18,19]

DIAGNOSIS

Antemortem diagnosis of ARF in horses is based on history, clinical signs, and laboratory findings of azotemia with concurrent isosthenuric or nearly isosthenuric urine.[2] Azotemia is a biochemical abnormality identified by abnormally high serum concentrations of urea nitrogen (SUN), creatinine (SCr), or more recently, symmetric dimethylarginine (SDMA). All of these measurements provide estimates of GFR, and all can increase from either intrinsic renal dysfunction or prerenal causes such as dehydration. SCr and SDMA levels are the preferred biochemical test in clinical practice for estimating GFR.[20,21] Both SCr and SDMA are freely filtered at the glomerulus and are expected to increase proportionally to the decrease in GFR but they might not increase above normal reference range until there is significant (approximately 75%) loss in GFR.[21] Because creatinine is formed in muscle, heavily muscled animals such as male Quarter horses and some Warmbloods may have physiologic SCr concentrations slightly above normal reference range. Serum urea nitrogen (SUN), also called blood urea nitrogen [BUN] generally provides a less accurate measurement of GRF than does SCr or SDMA.[22] Urea is reabsorbed from the glomerular filtrate in the renal tubules and resorption is increased with low urine flow rates as occurs during dehydration. Therefore, a SUN:SCr ratio has been proposed as a means of separating renal azotemia from prerenal azotemia. Although the concept seems reasonable, this is not a reliable test for separating the 2 conditions.[23] Urine creatine to SCr ratios can be helpful in differentiating prerenal and renal azotemia.[24]

The best and most practical routine laboratory test used to distinguish renal dysfunction/azotemia from prerenal azotemia is urine specific gravity (USG). The ability of the kidney to dilute or concentrate urine is lost when approximately two-thirds of tubular function is lost, and urine osmolarity will be comparable to serum osmolarity. Horses with ARF generally have a USG between 1.008 and 1.016, which corresponds to the osmolarity of serum and glomerular filtrate within Bowman capsule. Some horses with peracute RF and azotemia may have USG as high as 1.022.[24] This higher than expected value may be caused by an azotemic/glycemic increase in serum osmolarity, an increase in solutes (eg, glucose or protein) in the urine, or variations in individual nephron function that are yet to achieve a steady state USG. Regardless, if the azotemic horse has a USG greater than 1.025, prerenal azotemia is the most likely cause. USG measurement via refractometer provides a more accurate estimate of urine osmolarity than urine dipsticks.[22] It is important to remember that some degree of prerenal azotemia is often present in patients with ARF. Cytologic examination of the urine can be helpful when evaluating suspected ARF cases, because AKI is frequently associated with increased red blood cells and occasionally casts in the urine. High white blood cells in the urine may suggest an infectious/inflammatory cause of the AKI.

Serum electrolyte abnormalities are common in horses with ARF, with hyponatremia and hypochloremia being the most common abnormalities.[22] Serum potassium concentrations are variable in acutely azotemic horses but when elevated, ARF, prerenal azotemia, obstructive nephropathy and uroabdomen are potential causes. With oliguric or anuric ARF, serum potassium concentrations may occasionally be dangerously high (>5.5 mEq/L) and require specific medical treatment (glucose or bicarbonate) to decrease potassium concentrations. Potassium levels generally decrease quickly following fluid therapy with prerenal azotemia. If the potassium concentration remains high after rehydration in a horse with azotemia, primary renal dysfunction should be considered likely. Serum magnesium can be high with either renal or prerenal azotemia, and metabolic acidosis can occur from either severe renal dysfunction or predisposing diseases. Serum calcium can be increased in ARF, although this is more commonly found with chronic renal failure.[25]

Renal biopsy should be considered if there is confusion as to etiology of the ARF or if additional prognostic information is needed. In this author's experience, biopsy results do not change management in the great majority of ARF cases. Renal biopsy is a relatively safe procedure if performed on the right kidney with ultrasound guidance. There are more complications reported with biopsy of the left kidney.[26] Visible hematuria is common after the biopsy, but this generally resolves within 48 hours. Colic may also occur after the biopsy, likely related to renal or perirenal hemorrhage.[26]

Ultrasound imaging of the kidneys with ARF from causes other than obstructive causes is often disappointingly normal. Some horses with ARF may have enlarged kidneys with widening of and a slight increase in echogenicity of the cortex (see Dr. Marta Cercone's article, "Imaging of the Urinary Tract," in this issue). Perirenal edema can be seen in some horses with ARF, and this is in this author's experience a poor prognostic finding.

TREATMENT OF ACUTE RENAL FAILURE

Treatment of ARF in horses can vary depending on cause and the practical or financial ability to provide treatments. An algorithm for possible treatment of ARF is provided (**Fig. 1**). The initial treatment for the majority of ARF cases should be treatment of any predisposing disorder (eg, sepsis, hemorrhage, or urinary obstruction) and correction of prerenal factors (dehydration and hypotension). All nephrotoxic drugs should be discontinued if possible. Fluid therapy is a first line of treatment in most cases. Crystalloids and vasopressors (if needed) are administered intravenously to normalize

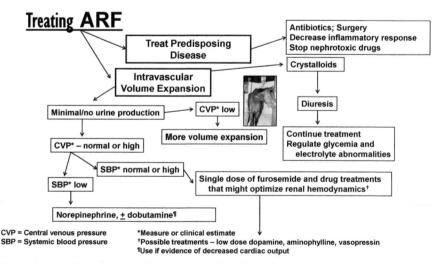

Fig. 1. An algorithm for possible treatment of ARF. The horse is the background is being treated for ARF with intravenous fluids while monitoring central venous pressure.

intravascular volume and blood pressure. Intravascular volume status can be estimated by clinical examination that specifically evaluates speed of jugular vein distention following manual occlusion, heart rate, and urine production, both before and after initiating fluid therapy. Ideally, central venous pressure (CVP) should be determined as a measurement of intravascular volume status, but this is rarely performed in the field. In a hospital setting, monitoring packed-cell volume (PCV) and plasma total solids concentration can provide important information regarding intravascular volume. Blood pressure measurements should also be performed if feasible. The optimal mean arterial pressure needed for preservation of renal function is reported to be in the 65 to 75 mm Hg range.[27] Measuring systemic blood pressure in the field is uncommon though, and indirect cuff measurements may not be accurate.[28,29] Therefore, palpation of arterial pulse pressure, noting mucosal capillary refill time and change in heart rate during fluid therapy can serve as means of estimating blood pressure. If the horse or foal urinates a moderate to large volume after receiving fluids, one can assume intravascular volume and systemic pressures are adequate for kidney function.

After correcting intravascular volume deficits and improving blood pressure, the next step in management of a horse with ARF is to determine if the patient has oliguric, anuric, or polyuric renal failure. Observing or ideally measuring urine production can determine this. Measurement of urine production should be performed in hospitalized neonatal foals. In older foals or adult horses, an observational estimate of urine production can be made. If the horse has not produced urine after an adequate fluid challenge, the bladder should be rectally palpated or visualized by ultrasound and the kidneys examined by ultrasound to rule out an obstructive nephropathy. If the initial fluid treatment and cardiovascular monitoring suggest oliguric or anuric ARF, CVP measurements should be initiated (see **Fig. 1**). It is critical that intravenous fluids are not given in excess to avoid abnormally high pressure in the venous circulation. If the venous pressure is high, harmful edema forms in tissues, including in and around the kidney, and abnormally high CVP inhibits venous return from the renal vein, further compromising renal function. CVP measurements are not always accurate, but if performed in the exact manner each time, noting the trend in pressure changes can help assess adequacy of fluid therapy. If the patient produces a large amount of urine following fluid therapy, treatment with fluids at approximately 2 times maintenance can continue while monitoring urine production, CVP, and SCr. Cardiac output measurements would be ideal in horses with oliguria and increased CVP, but this is difficult to perform in the field.[28,29] It is common, especially with nephrotoxic ARF, for horses to respond well to fluid therapy and quickly become polyuric, but SCr may not decrease significantly for 2 to 4 days. The establishment of polyuria following fluid treatments does not guarantee the GFR will improve, although the presence of polyuria is a good prognostic finding compared with oliguria or anuria. Serum electrolytes,acid-base and markers of GFR should be monitored throughout the treatment. Horses with polyuric ARF that are not eating because of uremia or a predisposing disease can develop hypokalemia and may require potassium supplementation. Potassium-containing fluids should be avoided in the initial fluid therapy for horses with ARF.

Historically, adult horses with polyuric ARF have been treated initially with a bolus of hypertonic saline followed by a continuous infusion of 0.9% saline, and in this author's experience, most cases have recovered, assuming the initiating disease could be treated successfully. Using hypertonic saline as an initial treatment in adult horses provides a practical way to rapidly increase intravascular volume, improve perfusion pressures, and quickly enhance urine production.[30] Increased urine production might improve renal function by flushing casts from partially obstructed tubules. This might be particularly helpful in horses with nephrotoxic or hypoxic tubular injury where casts are thought to commonly contribute to the decreased GFR. The administration of hypertonic saline can also quickly provide valuable information as to whether the horse has polyuric or oliguric/anuric renal failure. The use of high saline fluids in neonatal foals has been more limited, because high aldosterone levels occur in both sick and healthy foals and create concern about hypernatremia.[31] In human medicine, there has been an effort to discontinue high chloride fluid treatment in septic and ARF patients because of the concern for increased AKI and less favorable outcome in patients treated with high chloride fluids.[32] The precise mechanism for the AKI and lowered patient outcome is unknown but could be associated with a high chloride concentration at the macula densa causing constriction of the corresponding afferent arteriole.[33] A recent study did not find an association between high chloride fluid administration and renal prognosis,[34] and some nephrologists still consider saline fluids acceptable treatment for AKI as long as plasma chloride concentration is closely monitored.[35] Similar equine studies, comparing outcome following saline versus balanced crystalloid fluid treatment are not available. If high chloride fluids are used in the treatment of ARF, both serum chloride and bicarbonate should be monitored.

Horses with oliguric or anuric ARF are much more difficult to treat than those with polyuric ARF. Fluid therapy, although the gold standard for treating polyuric ARF, is of limited value in treating oliguric ARF beyond correcting intravascular volume deficits and hypotension. Continued large volume fluid treatments in oliguric/anuric patients can be harmful for reasons previously mentioned. Unless the oliguric patient can be converted to polyuria, the prognosis is poor, because renal replacement therapy is not widely available in horses. If fluid volume treatments are adequate to ensure normalization of intravascular volume, but limited or no urine has been produced, arterial blood pressure and cardiac output should be evaluated, as abnormalities in either might be adversely affecting renal function in spite of normal intravascular volume. If cardiac output or arterial pressures are thought to be abnormal, an attempt to correct these should be the next treatment. Dobutamine (in hopes of improving cardiac index) and norepinephrine (to normalize arterial pressures) are common treatments for these purposes in equine practice.[36] However, the ability of dobutamine to improve cardiac function in standing horses has recently been questioned.[37] If intravascular volume, arterial blood pressure, and cardiac output are adequate but the horse remains oliguric or anuric, an abnormality in intrarenal hemodynamics (functional or structural such as thrombosis) and/or tubular obstruction are likely causes for the oliguria/anuria. This is assuming a primary obstructive nephropathy is ruled out. At this point, there is a guessing game as to what drug, if any, might improve intrarenal dynamics such that GFR and urine production are increased. No single drug has proven effective in restoring GFR and urine production in large clinical studies in people with AKI.[38] The lack of an effective drug for treating oliguric ARF could be explained by the heterogeneous nature of the disease and disparate reasons for the renal dysfunction between patients.[38] It seems plausible that some drugs may have been effective in a small subset of patients in large clinical studies but not enough for statistical significance. So what does the equine clinician do when faced with a horse with oliguric or anuric ARF and increasing SCr after extrarenal (pre and post) mechanisms for disease are ruled out? One possibility is attempt to change intrarenal hemodynamics and tubular function with an unproven drug treatment. Perhaps the easiest and earliest treatment to try in hopes of causing polyuria is a single dose of furosemide, although studies in people have not found benefit in using furosemide in treating AKI.[39] Other drugs that could be used in an attempt to improve urine production and possibly GRF are fenoldopam, dopamine, theophylline/aminophylline, mannitol, alpha agonists, and norepinephrine. Fenoldopam mesylate is a selective dopamine receptor D_1 agonist, which induces vasodilation of the renal vessels. Low-dosage fenoldopam (0.04 μg/kg/min) significantly increased urine output but had no significant effect on creatinine clearance in a healthy foal study.[40] Dopamine at low doses (1–5 μg/kg/min) can stimulate renal dopamine receptors. In awake adult horses, low-dose dopamine caused renal vasodilation, increased renal blood flow, and increased urine production without systemic cardiovascular effects.[41] Although only an observation, this author has had occasional clinical success using low-dose dopamine to improve urine production and GRF in a small number of adult horses with oliguric renal failure. In some horses, the oliguria returned when dopamine was discontinued and then improved again when dopamine treatment was reinstated. In a recent publication on a horse with myoglobinuric ARF, infusion of micro doses of dopamine appeared effective in increasing urine production and decreasing serum levels of BUN and creatinine.[42] Aminophylline and mannitol are other drugs used in the treatment of ARF, but like dopamine and all the drugs discussed, strong evidence for their efficacy could not be found. Aminophylline and theophylline inhibits adenosine, a potent afferent arteriole vasoconstrictor, and this inhibition could improve GFR.[43] Aminophylline has been found to lower creatinine in pediatric patients with AKI but did not improve urine production or outcome.[43] This author has had some clinical success using aminophylline to treat oliguric ARF in neonates. Mannitol treatment for ARF is difficult to recommend, because it can cause severe osmotic injury to tubules.[44] Norepinephrine infusion (0.3 μg/kg/min) in healthy foals increased arterial blood pressure, systemic vascular resistance, urine output, and creatinine clearance.[45] I believe norepinephrine might currently be the preferred pressor drug for the treatment of foals with hypotension and ARF.

Horses and foals with persistent oliguria or anuria and no improvement in SCr after appropriate fluid therapy and therapeutic trials with one or more of the above listed drugs are candidates for renal replacement treatment. Renal replacement treatments performed in horses and foals with ARF include peritoneal dialysis, hemodialysis, and hemodiafiltration.[11,46,47,48] Peritoneal dialysis can be performed on horses with minimal or no special equipment, but the treatment is not very effective in removing uremic toxins or remaining toxic drugs.[49] Hemodialysis and hemodiafiltration require specialized equipment and in horses have only been performed short term.[11,46,48] The purpose of any dialysis treatment is to reduce circulating uremic and chemical toxins and to stabilize metabolic and fluid compartment abnormalities, providing more time for return of renal function.

Infectious causes of ARF in horses are uncommon, but leptospirosis should be considered in equines of all ages with ARF, fever, and pyuria without visible bacteriuria. Beta-lactam antibiotics or enrofloxacin are recommended treatments for equine leptospirosis.[18,19] If the SCr is greatly elevated, the antibiotic dosing interval might need to be prolonged to prevent exceeding high and potentially toxic serum levels of the antibiotics. Obstructive causes of ARF are mostly treated by surgical removal of the obstruction (see Dr. Susan L. Fubini's article, "Surgery for Uroperitoneum," in this issue).

PROGNOSIS OF ACUTE RENAL FAILURE

The prognosis for horses and foals with hemodynamically mediated nephropathy is often determined more by the ability to treat the primary disease (eg, septic shock or hemorrhage) than the degree of renal dysfunction itself. If the primary disease is successfully treated and the patient is producing adequate urine with a decrease in

SCr over the initial 24 to 72 hours of treatment, the prognosis is often good.[50] Prognostic considerations for nephrotoxic ARF include the amount of urine produced, stabilization of SCr in the first 48 hours of treatment, and the concentration of any nephrotoxic drug that may still be in systemic circulation or in the kidney. In many cases, fluid therapy may cause a modest decline in azotemia, but this could be caused by volume expansion alone, and only with a continual decline in SCr can the prognosis be favorable. Two to 4 days of fluid therapy may be necessary before SCr begins to decline following nephrotoxic ARF. Once SCr has declined to near-normal range, fluid therapy can usually be discontinued if the horse appears clinically normal. There is likely no reason for alarm if SCr increases 0.3 mg/dL ± after discontinuing intravenous fluid therapy, as this may just reflect a contraction of the intravascular volume. Continued monitoring of SCr is necessary to confirm that markers of GFR continue to normalize.

Horses and foals with oliguric or anuric renal failure have a guarded to poor prognosis, respectively. If the oliguria/anuria is converted to polyuria, then the prognosis improves, but unless there is a gradual decline in SCr to normal or near normal range, the prognosis remains guarded. Remember that a conversion from oliguria/anuria to polyuria does not guarantee an improvement in GFR, but it does makes continuation of standard medical treatment possible as opposed to renal replacement treatments.

Common sense suggests that extreme elevations in SCr or other markers of GFR would indicate a poor prognosis, but that is not always the case. This author treated 1 horse with vitamin K3-induced ARF that had an initial SCr of 21 mg/dL, and following 2 weeks of treatment, SCr was 1.7 mg/dL. Although a decline in SCr to near normal upper reference range can often occur within a week of initiating treatment for ARF, a final SCr concentration may not occur for 2 to 6 months after treatment. This is because, in response to loss of nephron function, less injured nephrons may hypertrophy, resulting in a gradual improvement in GFR and decrease in SCr concentration. This loss of function-gain of function relates to the heterogeneity of individual nephron disease following AKI. If the SCr or other markers of GFR return to normal or near-normal levels, that should indicate sufficient function for a relatively normal life span and athletic activity, but prevention of further kidney injury from medication or hypovolemia is important. Although are no statistics are available, it is this author's experience that stallions and mares that have stabilized SCr less than 3.2 mg/dL can usually maintain their reproductive status.

Routine ultrasound examination of the kidneys of most horses with ARF provides only modest information regarding prognosis. Perirenal edema might lower the prognosis, but some horses with perirenal edema survive ARF. Unexpected complications during treatment of ARF can negatively affect prognosis. Laminitis is not common in horses with ARF unless they also have colitis or systemic inflammatory disease, but it can occur without these predisposing disorders. If uremic encephalopathy develops, the prognosis is grave. Horses and foals with leptospirosis and ARF have a good prognosis with proper treatments.

Prognosis for acute obstructive nephropathy cases depends on rapid alleviation of the obstruction and correction of life-threating hyperkalemia if present.

PREVENTION OF ACUTE KIDNEY INJURY AND RENAL FAILURE

As an equine internist, I know how disheartening it can be when a patient develops ARF while being treated for another disease. Aminoglycosides and tetracycline are commonly used drugs that are high risk for causing AKI and even failure, and their risk increases if they are administered for a prolonged time or to a dehydrated or hypotensive patient. Therefore, it is imperative that the patient is properly hydrated prior to or soon after initiating treatment with any nephrotoxic drug. In field practice, clinical judgment will dictate which animals receive potentially nephrotoxic drugs prior to fluid therapy. High-risk patients that are persistently dehydrated, hypotensive, or hypoxemic should have SCr monitored closely when potentially nephrotoxic drugs are being used. If SCr increases 0.3 mg/dL or more, then the nephrotoxic drug should be withdrawn unless the drug is an essential treatment. In those cases, the drug could be continued if intermittent bolus or continual fluid therapy diuresis is performed ,and the interval of drug treatment is prolonged by the estimated percentage decrease in GFR. Drug monitoring (trough levels) of aminoglycosides is used to determine if toxic levels are being approached and as a guide to determine treatment interval. High calcium diets or intravenous administration of calcium to horses provides some protection against aminoglycoside toxicity.[51,52] Urinary enzymuria and urinary fractional excretion of sodium measurements could be used to detect early nephrotoxicity.[53] These are seldom used in practice, as they rarely provide clinically important information regarding renal function and may not have significant advantages over the close monitoring of SCr or SDMA.

Although NSAIDs rarely cause ARF, they can cause AKI, including interstitial nephritis, renal crest necrosis, tubular necrosis, and a decrease in glomerular perfusion.[54,55] Therefore, they should be used in appropriate doses and preferably in horses with normal hydration status. Their early use in ill horses with no pre-existing renal dysfunction is unlikely to cause functional renal problems. Selective and nonselective cyclooxygenase inhibitors could cause renal injury if used at high doses for prolonged periods or when administered to dehydrated horses.[54] Intravenously administered sodium bicarbonate and the resulting urine alkalization may provide some protection against pigment nephosis.[56] Renoprotection for horses with systemic inflammatory diseases and ill horses undergoing general anesthesia include maintenance of intravascular volume, systemic blood pressure, oxygenation; and prevention of fluid overload. Monitoring urine production and judicious use of nephrotoxic drugs are also important in the prevention of ARF. Although not studied in horses, alleviation of abnormally high abdominal pressure after abdominal surgery may improve hemodynamics to the kidney and urine flow, both of which might improve GFR and lessen the risk of tubular injury.[57]

SUMMARY

This article provided information on causes, diagnosis, treatment, and prevention of AKI and failure in horses and foals. Treatment guidelines based on a review of publications discussing equine and human ARF and this author's clinical experiences treating equines with acute renal failure are provided.

DISCLOSURE

The author has nothing to disclose.

REFERENCES

1. Savage VL, Marr CM, Bailey M, et al. Prevalence of acute kidney injury in a population of hospitalized horses. J Vet Intern Med 2019;33(5):2294–301.
2. Bayly WM. Acute renal failure. In: Reed SM, Bayly WM, Sellon DC, editors. Equine internal medicine. 4th edition. St.Louis (MO): Elsevier; 2018. 933–925.
3. Hilton R. Defining acute renal failure. CMAJ 2011;183(10):1167–9.

4. Geor RJ. Acute renal failure in horses. Vet Clin North Am Equine Prac 2007;23: 577–91.
5. Cotovio M, Monreal L, Armengo L, et al. Fibrin deposits and organ failure in newborn foals with severe septicemia. J Vet Intern Med 2008;22:1403–10.
6. Divers TJ, Whitlock RH, Byars TD, et al. Acute renal failure in six horses resulting from haemodynamic causes. Equine Vet J 1987;19(3):178–84.
7. Schott HC II. Review of azotemia in foals. 57th Annual Convention of the American Association of Equine Practitioners, 18-22 November 2011, San Antonio, (TX); 2011;328–34.
8. Roby KA, Reef VB, Shaw DP, et al. Rupture of an aortic sinus aneurysm in a 15-year-old broodmare. J Am Vet Med Assoc 1986;189:305–8.
9. Bartol JM, Divers TJ, Perkins GA. Nephrotoxicant-induced acute renal failure in five horses. Compcontin Educ Pract Vet 2000;22:870–6.
10. Sweilen WM. A prospective comparative study of gentamicin- and amikacin-induced nephrotoxicity in patients with normal baseline renal function. Fund Clin Pharmacol 2009;23:515–20.
11. Vivrette S, Cowgill LD, Pascoe J, et al. Hemodialysis for treatment of oxytetracycline-induced acute renal failure in a neonatal foal. J Am Vet Med Assoc 1993;203:105–7.
12. Krueger CR, Mitchell CF, Leise BS, et al. Pharmacokinetics and pharmacodynamics of clodronate disodium evaluated in plasma, synovial fluid and urine. Equine Vet J 2020;52:725–32.
13. Alward A, Corriher CA, Barton MH, et al. Red maple (*Acer rubrum*) leaf toxicosis in horses: a retrospective study of 32 cases. J Vet Intern Med 2006;20:1197–201.
14. Sprayberry KA, Madigan J, LeCouteur RA, et al. Renal failure, laminitis, and colitis following severe rhabdomyolysis in a draft horse-cross with polysaccharide storage myopathy. Can Vet J 1998;39:500–3.
15. Warner AF. Methemoglobinemia and hemolytic anemia in a horse with acute renal failure. Comp Cont Educ Pract Vet 1984;6:S465–8. S472.
16. el-Ashker MR. Acute kidney injury mediated by oxidative stress in Egyptian horses with exertional rhabdomyolysi. Vet Res Commun 2011;35:35.
17. Ribeiro PR, Bianchi MV, Henker LC, et al. Acute renal failure in a horse following bee sting toxicity. Ciencia Rural 2020;50(5):11.
18. Frellstedt L, Slovis NM. Acute renal disease from *Leptospira interrogans* in three yearlings from the same farm. Equine Vet Educ 2009;21:478–84.
19. Divers TJ, Byars TD, Shin SJ. Renal dysfunction associated with infection of Leptospira interrogans in a horse. J Am Vet Med Assoc 1992;201(9):1391–2.
20. Schott HC II, Gallant LR, Coyne M, et al. Symmetric dimethylarginine and creatinine concentrations in serum of healthy draft horses. J Vet Intern Med 2021;35: 1147–54.
21. Siwinska N, Zak A, Slowikowska M, et al. Serum symmetric dimethylarginine concentration in healthy horses and horses with acute kidney injury. BMC Vet Res 2020;16:396–402.
22. Schott HCI, Esser MM. The sick adult horse: renal clinical pathologic testing and urinalysis. Vet Clin North Am Equine Pract 2020;36:121–34.
23. Duncan JR, Prasse KW, Mahaffey EA. Veterinary laboratory medicine. 3rd edition. Iowa City, (IA): Iowa State University Press; 1994. p. 180.
24. Grossman BS, Brobst DF, Kramer JW, et al. Urinary indices for differentiation of prerenal azotemia and renal azotemia in horses. J Am Vet Med Assoc 1982; 180:284–8.

25. LeRoy B, Woolums A, Wass J, et al. The relationship between serum calcium concentration and outcome in horses with renal failure presented to referral hospitals. J Vet Intern Med 2011;25(6):1426–30.

26. Tyner GA, Nolen-Walston RD, Hall T, et al. A multicenter retrospective study of 151 renal biopsies in horses. J Vet Intern Med 2011;25:532–9.

27. Suarez J, Busse LW. New strategies to optimize renal haemodynamics. Curr Opin Crit Care 2020;26:536–42.

28. Heliczer N, Lorello O, Casoni D, et al. Accuracy and precision of noninvasive blood pressure in normo-, hyper-, and hypotensive standing and anesthetized adult horses. J Vet Intern Med 2016;30:866–72.

29. Shih AC. Cardiac monitoring in horses. Vet Clin N Am Equine Pract 2019;35:205–21.

30. Crabtree NE, et al, Crabtree NE, Epstein KL. Current concepts in fluid therapy in horses. Front Vet Sci 2021;29:648774.

31. Hollis AR, Boston RC, Corley KT. Plasma aldosterone, vasopressin and atrial natriuretic peptide in hypovolaemia: a preliminary comparative study of neonatal and mature horses. Equine Vet J 2008;40:64–9.

32. Yunos NM, Bellomo R, Glassford N, et al. Chloride-liberal vs. chloride-restrictive intravenous fluid administration and acute kidney injury: an extended analysis. Intensive Care Med 2015;41:257–64.

33. Rein JL, Coca SG. I don't get no respect": the role of chloride in acute kidney injury. Am J Physiol-renal Physiol 2019;316:F587–605.

34. Chapalain X, Huet O, Balzer T, et al. Does chloride intake at the early phase of septic shock resuscitation impact on renal outcome. Shock 2021;56(3):425–32. Online ahead of print.

35. Gameiro J, Fonseca JA, Outerelo C, et al. Acute kidney injury: from diagnosis to prevention and treatment strategies. J Clin Med 2020;9:1704–25.

36. Craig CA, Haskins SC, Hildebrand SV. The cardiopulmonary effects of dobutamine and norepinephrine in isoflurane-anesthetized foals. Vet Anaesth Anal 2007;34:337–87.

37. Meier M, Bettschart-Wolfensberger R, Schwarzwald CC, et al. Effects of dobutamine on cardiovascular function and oxygen delivery in standing horses. J Vet Pharmacol Ther 2020;43:470–6.

38. Moore PK, Hsu RK, Liu KD. Management of acute kidney injury: core curriculum. Am J Kidney Dis 2018;72:136–48.

39. Power BM. Benefits and risks of furosemide in acute kidney injury. Anaesth 2010;283–93.

40. Hollis AR, Ousey JC, Palmer L, et al. Effects of fenoldopam mesylate on systemic hemodynamics and indices of renal function in normotensive neonatal foals. J Vet Intern Med 2006;20:595–600.

41. Trim CM, Moore JN, Clark ES. Renal effects of dopamine infusion in conscious horses. Equine Vet J 1989;21:124–8.

42. Matsuda H, Matsuda K, Muko R, et al. Short-term infusion of ultralow-dose dopamine in an adult horse with acute kidney injury: a case report. Vet Anim Sci 2021; 112:100176.

43. Alsaadoun S, Rustom F, Hassan HA, et al. Aminophylline for improving acute kidney injury in pediatric patients: a systematic review and meta-analysis. Int J Health Sci 2020;14:44–51.

44. Nomani AZ, Nabi Z, Rashid H, et al. Osmotic nephrosis with mannitol: review article. Ren Fail 2014;36:1169–76.

45. Hollis AR, Ousey JC, Palmer L, et al. Effects of norepinephrine and combined norepinephrine and fenoldopam infusion on systemic hemodynamics and indices of renal function in normotensive neonatal foals. J Vet Intern Med 2008;22: 1210–5.
46. Fouche N, Graubner C, Lanz S, et al. Acute kidney injury due to *Leptospira interrogans* in 4 foals and use of renal replacement therapy with intermittent hemodiafiltration in 1 foal. J Vet Intern Med 2020;34:1007–12.
47. Gallatin LL, Couetil LL, Ash SR. Use of continuous-flow peritoneal dialysis for the treatment of acute renal failure in an adult horse. J Am Vet Med Assoc 2005;226: 756–9.
48. Wong DM, Ruby RE, Eatroff A, et al. Use of renal replacement therapy in a neonatal foal with postresuscitation acute renal failure. J Vet Intern Med 2017; 31:593–7.
49. Sweeney RW, MacDonald M, Hall J, et al. Kinetics of gentamicin elimination in two horses with acute renal failure. Equine Vet J 1988;20:182–4.
50. Groover ES, Woolums AR, Cole DJ, et al. Risk factors associated with renal insufficiency in horses with primary gastrointestinal disease: 26 cases (2000–2003). J Am Vet Med Assoc 2006;228(4):572–7.
51. Brashier MK, Geor RJ, Ames TR, et al. Effect of intravenous calcium administration on gentamicin-induced nephrotoxicosis in ponies. Am J Vet Res 1998;59: 1055–62.
52. Schumacher J, Wilson RC, Spano JS, et al. Effect of diet on gentamicin-induced nephrotoxicosis in horses. Am J Vet Res 1991;52:1274–8.
53. Rossier Y, Divers TJ, Sweeney RW. Variations in urinary gamma glutamyl transferase/urinary creatinine ratio in horses with or without pleuropneumonia treated with gentamicin. Equine Vet J 1995;27:217–20.
54. Read WK. Renal medullary crest necrosis associated with phenylbutazone therapy in horses. Vet Pathol 1983;20:662–9.
55. Raidal SL, Hughes KJ, Charman AL, et al. Effects of meloxicam and phenylbutazone on renal responses to furosemide, dobutamine, and exercise in horses. Am J Vet Res 2014;75:668–79.
56. Lalich JJ, Schwartz SI. The role of aciduria in the development of hemoglobinuric nephrosis in dehydrated rabbits. J Exp Med 1950;92:11–23.
57. Scholz H, Bolvin FJ, Schmidt-Ott KM, et al. Kidney physiology and susceptibility to acute kidney injury: implications for renoprotection. Nat Rev Nephrol 2021;17: 335–49.

Chronic Renal Failure-Causes, Clinical Findings, Treatments and Prognosis

Emil Olsen, DVM, PhD[a],*, Gaby van Galen, DVM, PhD[b,1]

KEYWORDS

• Chronic kidney disease • Chronic renal failure • Horse • Kidneys

KEY POINTS

• The most common clinical signs of CKD are weight loss, polyuria/polydipsia, and ventral edema.
• Glomerular filtration rate is the reference standard for evaluating kidney function and can be obtained by iohexol clearance time.
• Creatinine is only elevated when approximately 75% of the nephrons are dysfunctional.
• CKD is a progressive and irreversible inflammatory and fibrosing process lasting over 3 months.
• Staging chronic kidney disease is helpful to assess severity, interventions, prognosis, and progression.

Abbreviations	
CKD	chronic Kidney Disease
GFR	glomerular Filtration Rate
AKI	acute Kidney Injury
UPC	urine-Protein to Urine-Creatinine Ratio
SDMA	symmetric Dimethylarginine
NGAL	neutrophil Gelatinase-Associated Lipocalin

CHRONIC KIDNEY DISEASE AND CHRONIC RENAL FAILURE-TERMINOLOGY

Chronic kidney disease (CKD) is a chronic, irreversible progressive disease of the kidneys, with a duration greater than 3 months. This encompasses multiple different renal

[a] Veterinary Teaching Hospital (Universitetsdjursjukhuset, UDS), Swedish Veterinary Agricultural University (SLU), Box 7040, Uppsala 75007, Sweden; [b] Equine Internal Medicine, University of Sydney, B01 - J.D. Stewart Building, Sydney, Australia
[1] Present address: Wallstrasse 2, Wallerfangen 66798, Germany.
* Corresponding author.
E-mail address: eo@sund.ku.dk
Twitter: @_Mr__E (E.O.)

Vet Clin Equine 38 (2022) 25–46
https://doi.org/10.1016/j.cveq.2021.11.003
0749-0739/22/© 2021 Elsevier Inc. All rights reserved.

diseases. In human and small animal literature, the term chronic renal failure has, for the past 20 years, been replaced with CKD, because the word failure reflects an end stage where the kidney function is impaired to a point where the patient cannot survive without kidney transplantation or dialysis. Renal disease can, however, be chronic without being end stage or even without functional loss. Therefore, the term CKD is believed to be more appropriate, and the authors have elected to follow the human terminology and apply this to equine medicine.

CKD is typically defined as functional or structural where both are the result of a chronic reduction in the glomerular filtration rate (GFR). Structural renal disease can be palpated or imaged, whereas functional kidney disease often has no or few palpatory or ultrasound changes. Structural disease (or damage) usually precedes alterations in function and can occur without loss of function or with loss of function based on the extent of the disease.

PREVALENCE

In horses, CKD is uncommonly reported in the literature and has until now received little scientific attention despite being regularly encountered in equine practice with a profound effect on patient health and quality of life. One retrospective study[1] looked at admissions to a referral hospital in North America and found an overall prevalence of CKD of 0.12% over a 32-year period. Horses over 15 years of age had an increased risk with a 0.23% prevalence, and in particular, stallions over 15 years of age, had a prevalence of 0.51%. Similarly, the prevalence of CKD increases with age in dogs,[2] cats,[3] and people.[4] This is suggested to be related to a decrease in GFR with increasing age, possibly because of irreversible damage to the nephrons accumulating over time. Similarly, this decrease in GFR was shown in horses.[5]

As a contrast, however, acute kidney injury (AKI) is a lot more common, with a prevalence of 14.8% in a recent study[6] of horses in a referral population, 23% of horses with colic presenting to a referral hospital (unpublished data, van Galen, 2021), and in 14.3% to 25.3% (depending on the method used for analysis) of neonatal foals in a Scandinavian referral population.[7]

DIAGNOSIS: CLINICAL FINDINGS

The clinical signs of CKD are not pathognomonic, but relatively nonspecific and reflect the degree of reduction in renal function. Often, patients are only recognized to have CKD when alterations in serum electrolytes, protein, or biomarkers of kidney function show up as incidental changes in screening blood tests, perhaps presenting with minor or none of the classic clinical signs.

The most-reported clinical sign of CKD in horses is weight loss (86%), followed by polyuria/polydipsia (56%) and ventral edema (42%).[1] Less common clinical signs are declining athletic performance, poor appetite, dull hair coat, uremic oral ulcerations, gastrointestinal ulceration, gingivitis, dental tartar, and changes in mentation and mild diarrhea.[8] Urinary changes, such as hematuria, can, in rare instances be noticed in horses with CKD.[9-11] Additionally, hypertensive cardiomyopathy has been described in 5 horses with CKD.[12]

Neurologic signs have been reported in horses with uremic encephalopathy, resulting in ataxia, paresis, forebrain signs with obtundation and head pressing, and anxiety and changes in cognition.[13] In people, uremic encephalopathy has been reported to show bilaterally symmetric MRI changes in the basal nuclei consistent with a toxic injury.[14] The pathogenesis of uremic encephalopathy is poorly understood, and it is currently not known which molecules cause the clinical neurologic signs.

DIAGNOSIS: LABORATORY FINDINGS

Azotemia or uremia is often encountered in blood samples. However, before jumping to a conclusion of renal disease, one must understand that azotemia is used as an umbrella term for abnormally increased concentrations of urea, creatinine, and other nonprotein nitrogenous substances in the blood. Azotemia is not synonymous with uremia that results from loss of kidney function, nor is it from chronic loss of renal function (vs acute loss). It is, therefore, possible to have azotemia without kidney disease, and it is important to differentiate prerenal (decreased perfusion [eg, dehydration, hypovolemic shock, or cardiac failure]), renal (decreased GFR caused by renal injury), or postrenal causes of azotemia (failure of excretion of nitrogenous waste such as obstruction of the urinary tract or rupture of the urinary bladder). Prerenal causes for azotemia are often mentioned in equine literature; however, following human literature, pure prerenal causes may be rare. Most prerenal causes are closely linked or intertwined with inflammatory changes and/or toxic insults. For example, a horse presenting with acute colic and cardiovascular shock will also have systemic inflammatory response syndrome (SIRS) and, at its most vulnerable moment, receive nephrotoxic drugs (flunixin and gentamicin are the most common nephrotoxic drugs administered to horses undergoing exploratory laparotomy). Such a high-risk patient with SIRS and hypovolemia, therefore, has compromised perfusion and inflammatory and toxic insults to the kidney. In addition, there is a continuum between prerenal and renal azotemia, where perfusion issues, if severe enough and present for long enough, will lead to intrinsic renal damage. Once determined that the azotemia is renal in nature, it should be determined if the changes are acute, acute-on-chronic, or chronic based on duration. It is imperative to note, that CKD is also possible without azotemia (eg, in unilateral chronic disease where the second kidney can compensate for the loss of function of 1 kidney).

Further laboratory assessment of kidney function can be performed on 3 levels: GFR, presence of proteins in the urine, and increased blood pressure.

Estimation of Glomerular Filtration Rate

Urea is the main waste product excreted in the urine, from protein catabolism, and is filtered by the glomerulus. Urea is reabsorbed in the proximal tubules and is therefore not a great marker of GFR; although a decrease in GFR may increase blood urea, it may also be increased from protein catabolism.

Creatinine has traditionally been used as an indicator of GFR, as it is produced in the muscle from creatine and filtered unhindered in the glomeruli. When GFR goes down, serum creatinine increases. Unfortunately, by the time creatinine is increased above reference range (**Fig. 1**), approximately 60% to 75% of the functional nephrons are lost,[15] and therapeutic interventions are therefore often too late. Serum creatinine varies markedly between individuals and with age and breed, such as higher in some normal quarter horses[16] with greater muscle mass and lower in cachexic animals with subnormal muscle mass. However, the variation within an individual is low, which makes it a good candidate to follow changes in renal function over time. If creatinine is increased above the reference range, it can be used as an estimate of disease progression and followed over time.[17] In early renal disease, a small increase in serum creatinine concentration indicates a large decrease in GFR, whereas in advanced renal disease a large increase indicates smaller changes in GFR.

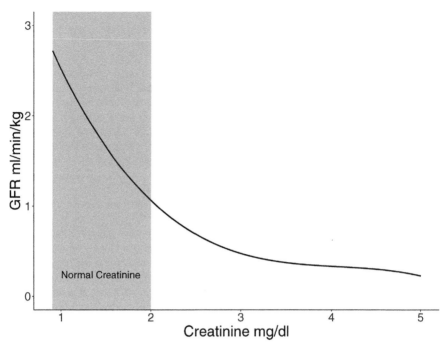

Fig. 1. The relationship between changes in blood creatinine and GFR. The figure illustrates that large decreases in GFR in early stages of CKD is accompanied by small increases in creatinine within the reference interval and could therefore be missed on routine bloodwork. In more advanced CKD with lower GFR, there is a marked increase in creatinine concentration not reflecting the level of change in glomerular function. (*Created with* data from Lippi and colleagues,[5] with fictive data added for creatinine over 2.0. *Inspired by* the IRIS Web site; www.iris-kidney.com.)

Therefore, small increases in creatinine are of limited clinical relevance in patients with CKD (see **Fig. 1**), whereas they are important in AKI.

The reference standard for assessment of glomerular function is to obtain an estimate of GFR by measuring the clearance of a substrate from the kidneys. Multiple

Table 1
Glomerular filtration rate changes for people as a reference standard for chronic kidney disease staging and prognostication[4] and comparative considerations for how categories could look in horses based on Lippi et al.[5]

GFR Category	GFR in % of Normal	GFR in People[1] mL/min/1.73 m²	GFR in Horses[2] ≤ 14 y[3]	GFR in Horses[2] ≥ 20 y[4]
Normal or high GFR	100%	≥ 90	≥ 2.0	≥ 2.1
Mildly decreased GFR	67%	60	1.3	1.4
Moderately decreased GFR	50%	45	1.0	1.1
Severely decreased GFR	33%	30	0.67	0.69
Kidney failure	17%	< 15	< 0.33	< 0.35

[1] mL/min/1.73 m².
[2] mL/min/kg.
[3] ≤ 14 y of age with serum creatinine < 1.5 mg/dL.
[4] ≥ 20 year old with serum creatinine < 1.5 mg/dL.

substrates have been used for this including inulin and iohexol.[18,19] For dogs, iohexol clearance has been shown to accurately diagnose CKD and detect change before the onset of azotemia.[19] Studies have evaluated iohexol clearance in horses and found it to be repeatable with a decreasing GFR estimate for horses over 20 years of age with increased creatinine.[5,20] **Table 1** is an illustration of how GFR is assessed in people and how a similar system could look for horses. This method of assessing GFR is rarely used for equine clinical cases, but could be implemented in chronic weight loss diagnostic work-ups with normal renal biomarkers.

Formulas exist in the literature to estimate GFR via creatinine clearance.[15] However, a recent study in cats attempted to develop a formula for GFR and found it to be highly inaccurate.[21] Therefore, this approach to estimate the GFR cannot be recommended without evidence in equine medicine.

In addition to estimating GFR, creatinine and urea concentrations can be used to calculate the urea to creatinine ratio. This ratio has been used as an estimator of renal function as both are freely filtered by the glomerulus, yet only urea's reabsorption is regulated. In a population of horses with CKD, 85% of the horses had increased urea to creatinine ratio greater than 10:1.[8] In a recent study in people, the urea to creatinine ratio was found to be unreliable to distinguish patients with prerenal AKI from patients with intrinsic AKI,[22] and another study found it to be a poor predictor of prerenal azotemia.[23]

Table 2
Rule of thumb guide for how to use urea nitrogen to creatinine ratio (urea:Cr) to determine if an injury is prerenal, renal, or postrenal

BUN	Creatinine	Location	Mechanism
↑↑	Normal	Prerenal	Urea nitrogen reabsorption is increased and therefore disproportionately elevated relative to creatinine; may be indicative of hypoperfusion; also, gastrointestinal bleeding or increased dietary protein can increase the ratio
Normal	Normal	Normal or postrenal	Normal or postrenal disease; urea nitrogen reabsorption is within normal limits
↓↓	Normal or increased	Renal	Renal damage causes reduced reabsorption of urea nitrogen, thus lowering the ratio; can also indicate liver disease (decrease urea formation) or malnutrition

Urinalysis

Cytology may be helpful in the initial evaluation where renal casts and renal tubular epithelial cells may be seen with tubular damage.[24] Erythrocytes and leukocytes, or even neoplastic cells can be found in the urine with some chronic renal diseases.

Loss of protein or albumin in the urine is common in CKD, but does not occur all the time. Evaluation of urine-protein to urine-creatinine ratio (UPC) is the reference standard to stage CKD in dogs and cats (IRIS; www.iris-kidney.com), and a similar ratio estimating the urine albumin to creatinine ratio is used in people combined with GFR measurement.[4] In people, a further distinction is made based on the amount of protein or albumin in the urine; mild elevations are named non-nephrotic proteinuria or microalbuminuria (incipient nephropathy); more pronounced losses in the urine are called nephrotic proteinuria or macroalbuminuria (clinical nephropathy). Albuminuria in people is typically determined in 24-hour urine collections or in spot collections, and increases are confirmed in at least 2 or 3 samples in a timeframe of 3 to 6 months, especially when proteinuria is detected on a urine dipstick.[25] Trace positivity can be ignored, as the dipsticks are sensitive and will often be trace positive with alkaline urine, which is common in healthy horses.[15,25] A quantitative measure of albumin or protein:creatinine ratio is preferred over dipstick testing. Marked proteinuria is considered a hallmark of equine glomerulonephritis.[15,24]

Fractional excretion of electrolytes in the urine of horses is reviewed elsewhere.[15,24] Increased fractional excretion of phosphate may be compensatory in dogs to avoid hyperphosphatemia and could be an early indicator of CKD.[26]

Blood Analysis: Electrolytes

A horse with increased creatinine and hypercalcemia should be highly suspect for CKD. Further nonspecific findings in horses with CKD are electrolyte abnormalities such as hyponatremia, hypochloremia, hyperkalemia, and variable phosphorous concentrations, predominantly hypophosphatemia and mild metabolic acidosis.[15] Hypoalbuminemia and anemia are also common findings.[8,15]

Because any injury to the kidneys activates the renin-angiotensin-aldosterone system,[27] the disease will be even further progressed by blood pressure increases. Blood pressure often increases in people[28] and dogs and cats[29] with CKD. Blood pressure measurements are underutilized in horses, but are easily obtained from the tail base and are validated in the standing conscious horse.[30,31]

New Biomarkers of Kidney Injury

Symmetric dimethylarginine (SDMA) is produced in cells during proteolysis where a methyl group is added to the amino acid arginine and released into the circulation. SDMA is filtered and cleared up to 90% by the kidneys and does not change with muscle mass or age in dogs.[17] SDMA appears to detect naturally occurring CKD 10 months before serum creatinine increases in dogs and 17 months before increases in serum creatinine in cats.[32] This earlier detection suggests SDMA increases when a lower percentage of the kidney is dysfunctional compared to creatinine. However, SDMA was falsely positive in 32% of cases and performed no better than creatinine in the detection of CKD in dogs without clinical signs.[32]

An SDMA assay has been validated in 165 draft horses without kidney disease; no significant effect was found on age or weight, but the breed significantly influenced the measurements.[33] SDMA also correctly classified horses as having AKI in a study involving clinical cases.[34,35] However, clinical data are currently lacking on its usefulness in horses with CKD. Furthermore, it is unclear if SDMA offers any benefit once CKD has already led to increased creatinine levels.

Neutrophil gelatinase-associated lipocalin (NGAL) is a member of the family of lipocalin-binding proteins and is found in neutrophils and in many tissues throughout the body including the kidneys. NGAL is filtered through the glomeruli and completely reabsorbed in the proximal tubules of the normal kidney. With an injury to the proximal tubules, the reabsorption is decreased, making NGAL is a biomarker of tubular injury.[17] In addition to the GFR functional markers creatinine, urea, and SDMA, it can be advantageous to have structural markers, similar to clinical pathology of the liver that has markers for injury to bile ducts and hepatocytes. An assay for NGAL has recently been validated, and horses with elevated creatinine values have been demonstrated to have significantly higher serum NGAL concentrations.[36] NGAL can also be measured in urine and combined with creatinine as a ratio. Currently only enzyme-linked immunosorbent assays (ELISAs) are available, which require multiple samples to be run at the same time, and analysis is not currently offered in commercial laboratories.

In human medicine, lots of other functional or structural renal biomarkers are available; among the most well-known are cystatin C (CysC), B2 microglobin (B2-M), kidney injury molecule (KIM-1), and N-Acetyl-b-O-glucosaminidase (NAG). It is likely that in the future multipanels of structural and functional biomarkers will standardly be used.

DIAGNOSIS: STAGING

In human medicine, guidelines for determining and staging the degree of kidney disease are well established through the guidelines from Improving Global Outcomes in Kidney Disease (KDIGO).[4] In these guidelines, CKD is defined as abnormalities of kidney structure or function for over 3 months with implications for health and further classified or staged based on functional testing of the GFR and degree of albumin in the urine.[4] In canine and feline medicine, the International Renal Interest Society (IRIS; www.iris-kidney.com) has recommended guidelines for staging CKD based on measurements of serum creatinine, the protein level in urine, and blood pressure levels.

Early detection and interventions are important to slow down the speed of progression and the development of secondary changes such as hypertension, cardiovascular disease, and end-stage kidney failure.[28] For an overview of staging in small medicine and extrapolation to how a staging system for CKD could look in horses, see **Tables 2–5**. The impact of staging and early intervention in horses is currently not documented.

DIAGNOSIS: OTHER COMPLEMENTARY EXAMINATIONS

An initial attempt at determining the underlying cause of the kidney disease and screening for structural abnormalities should be initiated, even though they are rarely found in horses.

Diagnostic imaging is reviewed in detail elsewhere in this issue; however, it should be emphasized that ultrasound of the kidneys is excellent to detect structural abnormalities in the kidneys such as uroliths, hydronephrosis, and indicators of CKD such as poor corticomedullary definitions.

Renal biopsies may provide invaluable information about the underlying cause of CKD.

Indications for renal biopsies in human medicine vary among nephrologists, but commonly they include idiopathic nephritic and nephrotic syndromes, diagnosis of unknown primary lesions, and evaluation of renal masses[38] and unexplained or rapidly declining GFR.[28] There is, however, consensus around contraindications. Renal biopsy, in human nephrology, is not indicated for evaluation of non-nephrotic proteinuria, isolated glomerular hematuria, slowly progressive renal failure with a known etiology, uncontrolled severe hypertension, inability to cooperate, solitary kidney, and uncontrollable bleeding diathesis.[38] For horses, currently, no consensus exists over the indications and contraindications for renal biopsies.

In a retrospective multicenter study of ultrasound-guided renal biopsies in 151 horses,[39] 17 horses developed complications. Minor complications (13 of 151 horses) included mild hemorrhage, transient colic, or fever. Major complications (4 of 151 horses) included fatal outcomes following profuse hemorrhage (1 of 151

Table 3
2019 criteria for staging dogs and cats with chronic kidney disease (from IRIS; www.iris-kidney.com) and adapted criteria for how they could look for horses based on similar degrees of increase and 95% confidence interval described in 165 horses[33] with duration over 3 months

Stage		Dogs	Cats	Horses	Comments - from IRIS
Normal	Creatinine (μmol/l)	< 125	< 140	< 180	
	Creatinine (mg/dL)	< 1.4	< 1.6	< 2.0	
	SDMA (μg/dL)	< 18	< 18	< 14	
1	Creatinine (μmol/l)	< 125	< 140	< 180	Normal blood creatinine or normal or mild increase blood SDMA; some other renal abnormalities are present (such as inadequate urinary concentrating ability, abnormal renal palpation or renal imaging, increasing blood creatinine or SDMA concentrations in samples collected serially)
	Creatinine (mg/dL)	< 1.4	< 1.6	< 2.0	
	SDMA (μg/dL)	< 18	< 18	< 14	
2	Creatinine (μmol/l)	125–250	140–250	180–250	Normal or mildly increased creatinine, mild renal azotemia (lower end of the range lies within reference ranges for creatinine for many laboratories, but the insensitivity of creatinine concentration as a screening test means that patients with creatinine values close to the upper reference limit often have excretory failure); mildly increased SDMA; clinical signs are usually mild or absent
	Creatinine (mg/dL)	1.4–2.8	1.6–2.8	2.0–3.0	
	SDMA (μg/dL)	18–35	18–25	14–30	
3	Creatinine (μmol/L)	251–440	251–440	251–450	Moderate renal azotemia; many extrarenal signs may be present, but their extent and severity may vary; if signs are absent, the case could be considered as early stage 3, while the presence of many or marked systemic signs might justify classification as late stage 3
	Creatinine (mg/dL)	2.9–5.0	2.9–5.0	3.1–5.0	
	SDMA (μg/dL)	36–54	26–38	31–45	
4	Creatinine (μmol/L)	> 440	> 440	> 450	Increasing risk of systemic clinical signs and uremic crisis
	Creatinine (mg/dL)	> 5.0	> 5.0	> 6.0	
	SDMA (μg/dL)	> 54	> 38	> 45	

Local laboratory establishment of reference ranges of serum creatinine can lead to different cut-off levels, and they might also slightly differ between breeds.

Table 4
Substaging of chronic kidney disease based on urine protein:creatinine value (from IRIS; www.iris-kidney.com) and adapted criteria for how they could look for horses with disease duration over 3 months, based on 24-h values in 11 horses[37]

Urine Protein: Creatinine ratio[1]			
Dogs	Cats	Horses	Substage
< 0.2	< 0.2	< 0.2	Nonproteinuric
0.2–0.5	0.2–0.5	0.2–0.5	Borderline proteinuric
> 0.5	> 0.4	> 0.5	Proteinuric

horses), obstructive blood clot in the bladder, abortion, and abdominal discomfort. In 72% of cases, there was agreement between biopsy and postmortem diagnosis. Complication rates were greater for biopsies of the left kidney (because of greater depth and poorer percutaneous accessibility) and horses with neoplasia of the kidney.[39]

In human nephrology, it is described that hypertension caused by CKD is a risk factor for bleeding complications following renal biopsy.[40,41] Therefore, the authors strongly recommend measuring blood pressure in equine patients before the renal biopsy procedure. In the previously mentioned equine study, automated biopsy guns, and manual Tru-cut needles were used and complication rates of 10% (4/40) and 15% (7/47) were reported, respectively. The techniques were not showing significantly different complication rates. However, in people, the use of automated biopsy guns (vs a manual Tru-cut biopsy instrument) results in fewer bleeding complications and produces biopsy samples with more glomeruli.[42] The authors believe that automated biopsy guns are therefore also the recommended biopsy tool in equine medicine.

The number of renal biopsies (3 to 4 biopsy passes vs 2 biopsy passes) do not influence complication rates in people.[41] It is currently unknown if this has an effect on horses. Renal biopsy should be performed under ultrasonographic guidance, and from areas that ultrasonographically shows structural lesions, avoiding large blood vessels. Also, one should aim at sampling from the cortex and the medulla.

Human biopsy samples are commonly submitted for light microscopy (H&E, PAS, silver methenamine, and trichrome stains), immunohistochemistry (eg, immunoglobins and their subclasses, complement components, fibrin, and virus identification), and electron microscopy (EM) investigation.[43] In human nephrology, EM was absolutely necessary to make a correct diagnosis in 21% of cases and resulted in clinical refinement of or addition to the diagnosis in another 24% of cases.[43] EM has been described

Table 5
Using blood pressure to substage for chronic kidney disease (from IRIS; www.iris-kidney.com) for dogs and cats. Adapted to standing horses with a duration of over 3 months, based on 2 experimental studies[30,31]

Systolic Arterial Blood Pressure mm Hg		Blood Pressure Substage	Risk of Future Target Organ Damage
Dog/Cat	Horse		
< 140	< 150	Normotensive	Minimal
140–159	150–169	Prehypertensive	Low
160–179	170–189	Hypertensive	Moderate
> 179	> 189	Severely Hypertensive	High

in canine and feline renal biopsy and was also considered an essential method for diagnosis and prognosis.[44] EM is not yet commonly applied in equine medicine.

PATHOGENESIS: ACUTE AND CHRONIC KIDNEY DISEASE ARE INTERLINKED

In human nephrology, it is well documented that patients with AKI often progress to CKD, and some patients have events of acute-on-chronic disease when they present to the hospital for AKI.[45,46] In recent years it has been documented that CKD is a risk factor for AKI, where the chronic disease process results in oscillating inflammation and fibrosis or what can be characterized as multiple acute episodes.[47,48] Indeed, this also appears to be the case in small animals,[48,49] and is most likely also happening to horses.

Three structural units can be injured in the kidney: the glomerulus, the tubulointerstitium, and the vasculature. The tubules are most commonly injured in AKI. After an injury to tubular cells, they activate a proinflammatory response and undergo apoptosis. Macrophages are initially activated during this phase in a proinflammatory (M1) mode. Pericytes are normally located near endothelial cells and migrate to the tubules to support regeneration in acute and chronic kidney disease. After the initial acute inflammatory response, the tubular cells appear stuck in the proinflammatory and profibrotic stages leading to CKD and scarring.[50] Macrophages switch to repair and fibrosis mode (M2) and sometimes stay in this repair mode, contributing to tubular fibrosis as shown in **Figs. 2** and **3**.[47] When the extracellular matrix is replaced with normal and abnormal (fibrosed and disorganized) tissue, filtration and structure of

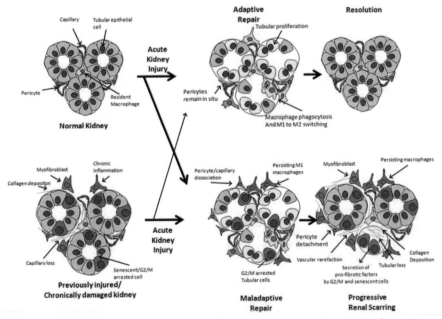

Fig. 2. A kidney with CKD is less likely to undergo complete adaptive repair after an acute renal insult. In the context of preinjury fibrosis, senescence, and microvascular loss the kidney is more likely to repair maladaptively with increased tubular loss and scarring. Although a normal kidney can respond to injury with adaptive repair, it is also recognized that with greater levels of injury and increasing age, maladaptive repair to CKD is more likely. (*From* Ferenbach and Bonventre[47].)

the nephron are lost.[51] After the initial adaptive repair and replacement of the extracellular matrix with dysfunctional units, tubular microvasculature is lost, and a resulting chronic low-grade hypoxia affects the entire kidney, leading to loss of glomeruli and subsequently increased filtration in the remaining glomeruli with increased oxygen consumption, leading to a vicious cycle of worsening renal hypoxia and further cell damage.[47]

Case example. Chronic Kidney Disease in a horse with suspected immun-mediated glomerulonephritis.

Case example. A 3-year-old thoroughbred gelding presented to the Cornell Equine and Nemo Farm Animal Hospital for lethargy and weight loss over the past 2 months. The horse had been treated multiple times intravenously with heterologous stem cells for tendinopathy. Clinical pathology suggested CKD with protein-losing nephropathy. The suspected etiology was immune-mediated glomerulonephritis. Membranoproliferative glomerulonephritis was confirmed based on postmortem histopathology of the kidney. The CKD occurred after the treatment with stem cells, but no proof of an association could be made.

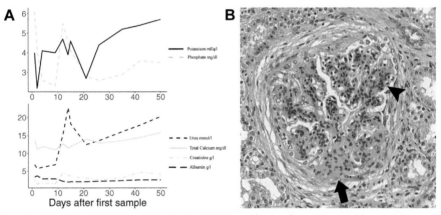

Fig. 3. (A) (plot). (B) (histopathology). (A) Changes in relevant serum parameters over 50 days in a horse with CKD from glomerulonephritis. Albumin RR: 3.0-3.7 g/L, total calcium RR: 10.9-12.8 mg/dL, phosphate RR: 2.1-4.2 mg/dL, creatinine 0.6-1.6 mg/dL, potassium RR: 2.6-4.5 mEq/L, and urea RR: 5.6-12.6 mmol/L. Note the acute exacerbation between days 10 and 15 improved with fluid therapy and the steady incline in urea and total calcium as well as slow incline in creatinine, potassium, phosphate, and total calcium. Urine protein level from a dipstick (not shown here) was ++, and urine-specific gravity was 1.010 (RR 1.012–1.040). Based on the staging that is proposed in this article, this horse would have suffered from stage 3 CKD with creatinine at 4.8 to 4.1 on the last two measurements. No blood pressure was obtained. (B) Histopathology picture from the horse in (A). Membranoproliferative glomerulonephritis has histologic features of both proliferative glomerulonephritis, which is characterized by increased cellularity of the glomerulus (arrowhead), and membranous glomerulonephritis, which is characterized by hyaline thickening of glomerular capillary basement membrane (arrow). H&E stain. (Courtesy of Dr. M Jager, DVM, DACVP, AHDC and Prof. T. Divers, DVM, DACVIM, DACVECC, Department of Clinical Sciences, Cornell University, Ithaca, NY Cornell University.)

CAUSES OF CHRONIC KIDNEY DISEASE

Changes in renal function can be from a reduction in the glomerular blood flow and perfusion pressure, loss of normal glomerular function, and loss of tubular functions, and changes in renal structure. Renal damage are commonly from congenital or obstructive causes. **Fig. 3** shows causes of CKD reported in equine literature.

CKD is traditionally categorized into tubulointerstitial disease, glomerular disease, and end-stage renal disease based on renal biopsies and postmortem findings. However, as indicated in the previous discussion of pathophysiology, an injury to 1 part of the nephron may result in chronic changes to all parts of the nephron.

Chronic tubulointerstitial disease, also called chronic interstitial nephritis, was found to be the most common histopathologic findings on 63 of 151 renal biopsies in horses;[39] however, an earlier study reported 38 of 99 horses to have glomerulonephritis as the most common finding.[1] Hemodynamic, hypoxic, and inflammatory changes, such as systemic inflammatory response syndrome (SIRS), septicemia, anemia, and hypovolemia, can lead to an acute injury[52] with the pathophysiologic implications of scarring discussed previously,[47] resulting in chronic interstitial nephritis. Chronic interstitial nephritis may also be caused by AKI from a toxic insult to the proximal tubules. Some examples include phenylbutazone causing renal papillary crest necrosis,[53] aminoglycosides, bisphosphonates as reported in people[54,55] and anecdotally in horses, or metals such as mercury and lead[56] may lead to scarring of the tubules and may progress to CKD.

Glomerulonephritis is the most common among the causes of CKD in horses based on an early report[1] and the second most common pattern on renal biopsies.[39] **Box 1** shows histopathology and selected clinical pathology changes over a 50-day period from a horse with CKD. A primary cause of glomerulonephritis in horses is the deposition of antibodies to the glomerular basement membrane from antigen-antibody complexes following chronic infection with group C *Streptococcus spp,*[57] *Leptospira Pomona*[58,59] and equine infectious anemia virus,[60] as well as purpura hemorrhagica.[61] As described previously, glomerulonephritis can also occur secondary to AKI and tubulointerstitial disease.

Nephrolithiasis

The presence of nephroliths, whether obstructive or not, is suggestive of CKD, perhaps a result of, or leading to chronic inflammation and fibrosis.[62–64] In a retrospective study of urolithiasis, 18 of 68 horses were mares, and 50 were males with 21 of 50 being stallions and 29 of 50 geldings ranging in age from 7 months to 27 years with a mean of 10 years. In 15 of 68 horses, the uroliths were in the kidneys, and in 2 horses they were present in 1 kidney and bladder; another 2 horses had uroliths in the bladder and both kidneys.[9] Clinical findings are slightly different to other causes of CKD in that horses with nephrolithiasis at times present with colic, pollakiuria, stranguria, and hematuria in addition to the traditional clinical signs of CKD described previously.[9,63] One case of colic and peritonitis in a horse following rupture of the kidney has also been described.[65] Urolithiasis of the lower urinary tract is discussed elsewhere in this issue, but it should be mentioned that obstruction of the ureters or urethra may lead to AKI and hydronephrosis[66] with a subsequent CKD. Rectal palpation and ultrasonography are essential for diagnosis, and in fact, all horses with lower urinary tract urolithiasis should be investigated for CKD and receive an ultrasound of the kidneys to rule out the presence of nephroliths. Furthermore, recurrent lower urinary tract urolithiasis may also be caused by pyelonephritis,[67] and ultrasonography and/or a catheter-obtained urine sample for culture and cytology should be performed in all horses with urolithiasis. The pathophysiology of urolithiasis in horses is not well understood. The alkaline urine and the large excretion of calcium carbonate in urine from horses[68] likely predispose to calcium carbonate uroliths in horses.[69] There is no evidence for choice of treatment in horses with urolithiasis. In small animals, the recommendation

Box 1
Etiologies of chronic kidney disease in horses based on the vitamin D system split into structural and functional causes

	Structural	Functional
Vascular		Infarcts
Inflammatory		Glomerulonephritis[1]
		Purpura hemorrhagica[61]
Infectious		Glomerulonephritis[1]
		Pyelonephritis[67]
		Leptospirosis[58,59]
		Streptococcus spp[57]
		Equine Infectious Anemia virus[60]
Toxic		Tubular necrosis with ischemic or toxic injury to the tubules: NSAIDS Aminoglycosides Oxytetracyclines Bisphosphonates Vitamin D supplementation Vitamin K3 (menadione), Lead Mercury
Traumatic		Trauma
Anomaly	Renal agenesis/contralateral obstruction and hydronephrosis Renal hypoplasia[85] Renal dysplasia[86,87] Polycystic kidney disease[88,89]	
Metabolic	Nephrolithiasis[9,62,63,65,66,72,90] Ureterolithiasis[9,62,63]	Hypertension[12]
Idiopathic		Chronic interstitial nephritis[1]
Neoplastic		Primary: renal carcinoma[82] Primary: renal adenocarcinoma[91] Primary: neuroendocrine tumors[92] Primary: nephroblastoma[83] Metastatic: lymphoma Metastatic: hemangiosarcoma[93] Metastatic: melanoma
Nutrition	Vitamin D	Vitamin D Toxicity (ingestion of Cestrum diurnum, wild jasmine)
	Plants	Sorghum, Oxalate containing plants, oak (flowers, leave buds or Acorn)[105]
Degenerative		End-stage kidney disease

is to attempt medical management including stimulating diuresis, and this is achieved in small animal medicine with diets containing a minimum of 70% moisture.[70] This may be achieved in horses with habituation to markedly watery mashes and grass as well as soaked hay. Liaising with an equine nutritionist might facilitate a slightly less alkaline pH of the urine, thereby reducing the rate of new urolith formation. Because pyelonephritis can be a predisposing factor,[9,67] a catheter-obtained urine sample for culture and cytology is recommended.

If medical management fails, the considerations for surgical management are progressive enlargement of the nephrolith, destruction of kidney tissue, and possible obstruction. Surgical management options in small animal medicine include percutaneous or endoscopic nephrolithectomy, nephrectomy, and in principle extracorporeal shockwave lithotripsy.[71] At least half of horses with nephrolithiasis have bilateral disease.[9,63,72] Lithotripsy has been successfully applied in a few horses.[73,74] Nephrectomy is a common surgical option used with unilateral disease.[73,75,76]

Pyelonephritis is a possible cause of CKD. It has been described in horses with urolithiasis,[9] recurrent urinary tract infections (mostly cystitis),[77] and lower motor neuron bladder or sorghum toxicity.[78] Pyelonephritis may even result in severe renal hemorrhage[10] (more information on urinary tract infections and pyelonephritis is available elsewhere in this issue). Therefore, it is recommended to perform bacterial culture for all horses with CKD and pyuria (or elevated leukocytes in the urine). If disease is unilateral, a urine sample can be obtained endoscopically directly from the ureter of the affected side.

End-stage renal disease is a disease stage, defined in human nephrology as fatal without dialysis and transplantation and a GFR less than 15 mL/min/1.73 m.[2] Extrapolated to horses and based on body weight in kilograms, GFR for horses younger than 14 years of age with end-stage renal disease would be less than 0.33 mL/min/kg for most horses and older than 20 years less than 0.35 mL/min/kg.

The marked decrease in GFR can result in oliguria or anuria, fluid retention, and edema, hypertension, ventricular dysfunction,[79] and eventually death. Some cases will still present with polyuria, presumably caused by hypertrophy of several nephrons and increased perfusion pressure. In people, end-stage renal disease also leads to a marked dysfunction of the immune system and risk of severe infections.[80] For most horses, end-stage renal disease results in euthanasia. On gross pathology, end-stage renal disease is characterized by smaller than normal, pale (from fibrosis), firmer than normal with an irregular surface. On histopathology, the tubules are completely fibrosed, and there is no trace of the original etiology.[8]

Neoplasias occur as a cause of CKD in horses, with primary neoplasias being the most common, constituting 75% of renal neoplasias in a retrospective postmortem study.[81] The primary tumor types are renal carcinomas, renal adenomas, neuroendocrine tumors, and nephroblastomas.[81–84] For metastatic neoplasias, multicentric lymphoma is the most common, followed by melanoma and hemangiosarcoma.[81] As with any neoplastic disease, a thorough investigation for metastasis should be performed with a clinical examination including an oral examination and rectal examination. Additionally, hematology, biochemistry, thoracic radiographs, and abdominal ultrasound and local lymph node aspirates should be performed. Percutaneous ultrasound-guided biopsies with an automated biopsy instrument can be obtained and can confirm the diagnosis. If the tumor is primary, unilateral nephrectomy may result in remission if it has not metastasized.[82,83]

It is essential to use the appropriate diagnostic workup including a thorough history to identify possible toxic insults, clinical examination along with the previously mentioned biomarkers of CKD, and diagnostic imaging to establish the chronicity and possible etiology. Staging as described previously is helpful to identify severity and monitor progression.

THERAPEUTIC OPTIONS

Treatment of pyelonephritis is described elsewhere in this issue.

If renal biopsy identifies glomerulonephritis and postinfectious glomerulonephritis is likely, with the primary infection being resolved or controlled, immunosuppressive therapy should be instigated with dexamethasone 0.1 mg/kg intravenously or intramuscularly once daily for 3 to 5 days, followed by oral prednisolone 1 mg/kg twice daily for 2 weeks, then tapered with 25% to a level where the clinical effect is present. Worsening may happen if the prednisolone is tapered or if the primary infection is not

Table 6
Management suggestions for horses with chronic kidney disease for each of the stages. Based on chronic kidney disease (from IRIS; www.iris-kidney.com) and adapted to horses

Stage 1	Avoid toxic insults such as the use of NSAIDs, aminoglycosides, oxytetracycline, bisphosphonates, and vitamin D. If nephrotoxic drugs are unavoidable, use the lowest dose and shortest treatment duration, monitor creatinine, and perform urine cytology every 48 hours to look for casts during and several days after the treatment
	Keep plenty of freshwater available to satisfy any PU/PD
	Monitor trends in creatinine, and urine protein:creatinine ratio every 3 months to assess and detect possible progression. Other novel markers can be assessed too; however, it is unclear at this point how useful monitoring over time is.
	Is the horse hypertensive with systolic blood pressure > 170 mm Hg or has evidence of target organ disease[29]? Treat with angiotensin-converting-enzyme (ACE) inhibitors such as benazepril (1 mg/kg body weight orally), ramipril (0.8 mg/kg body weight orally).[29]
	If the urine protein:creatinine ratio is > 0.5, measured at least twice, measured 2 weeks apart: get the hay analyzed for nutritional contents and consult an equine nutritionist to reduce protein intake to a minimum sustainable level.[94]
	Monitor for hypercalcemia and hypophosphatemia. Keep calcium < 7.2 mg/dL / 1.8 mmol/L and phosphorus > 3.1 mg/dL / 1 mmol/L. Consult an equine nutritionist.
Stage 2	As stage 1 plus:
	Get the hay analyzed for nutritional contents and consult an equine nutritionist to reduce protein intake to a minimum sustainable level.
	Monitor potassium and if low, supplement with oral potassium (0.1–0.2 g/kg orally), or consult an equine nutritionist.
Stage 3	As stage 2 plus:
	Monitor for anemia. When Erythropoitin (EPO) is administered to horses, there is a risk for antibody production against EPO and further anemia.
	If inappetent, change to more palatable food and get the horse out on fresh grass. In severe cases, appetite-stimulating drugs can be tried.
	Subcutaneous fluids are used in dogs and cats, but the volume to inject is not feasible for at-home treatment of horses. Mash-spiked water or other ways of increasing water intake may be helpful. Horses with electrolyte derangements sometimes also enjoy drinking water with electrolytes, which can at the same time maintain fluid balance and correct electrolyte derangements.
Stage 4	As 3 plus:
	Monitor ionized calcium and keep Ca < 7.2mg/dL / 1.8mmol/L and monitor for hypophosphatemia and keep phosphorus > 3.1 mg/dL / 1 mmol/L. Monitor potassium and keep < 5 mmol/L / mEq/L. Adapt diet accordingly and consult an equine nutritionist. If hypercalcemic, avoid calcium-rich foods such as alfalfa hay.
	In dogs and cats, esophageal feeding tubes are considered at this stage; however, this is not usually feasible for horses outside the hospital.

under control or recurs. In some cases, concurrent antimicrobial treatment can be recommended.

As described previously, CKD is a progressive and irreversible condition, and as such the primary goal, once diagnosed and staged, is to manage the side effects of CKD, focusing on proteinemia, hypertension, electrolyte derangements, and nutrition.

An overview of management options for horses is summarized in **Table 6**. As described previously, nutritional management is key to managing CKD, with balanced and adapted protein level to avoid catabolism of muscles, low calcium hay, often switching away from alfalfa hay and focusing on low-salt diets and keeping sugar and carbohydrates below 1.5 g/kg to reduce the risk of gastric ulcers and adding omega-3 polyunsaturated fatty acids for the anti-inflammatory effect and weight gain.[95] It may be helpful to add vegetable oils to the food to increase caloric intake; start carefully with a maximum of 100 mL split into 2 times per day to reduce the risk of diarrhea. It is important that dietary changes not affect the horse's overall appetite, or else weight loss and clinical deterioration will be enhanced.

Vitamin E has been found to have beneficial effects in people and in mice with CKD, lowering ADMA levels (an endogenous inhibitor of endothelial nitric oxide synthase) and attenuating the progression of renal fibrosis.[96,97] Vitamin E is also recommended when oils are fed.

Many food supplements are on the market to support the kidneys in people and small animals; there is no scientific evidence of the benefit of any of these supplements in horses.

In people, regular exercise training generally is associated with improved health outcomes in individuals with CKD.[98,99] It is likely that mild regular exercise of horses might have a similar effect.

The standard of care in human nephrology is to instigate renal replacement therapy (dialysis) once the GFR is severely reduced (approximately stage 4 in the IRIS staging system).[4] Other indicators of renal replacement therapy are uncontrolled hypertension, anemia requiring erythropoietin treatment or severe electrolyte, and acid-base derangements. Renal replacement therapy has been described in a foal with postresuscitation AKI.[100] Peritoneal dialysis can be used as a cheaper alternative and has been described in horses with AKI but is not sustainable for CKD.[101–103]

Novel therapeutics under development for people target the progressive fibrosing of the renal tubules by arresting the epithelial cell differentiation, nephroprotective epigenetic modulators and the targeting of growth factors contributing to fibrosis in kidney disease.[104]

The prognosis for long-term survival is poor in horses; however, it may be possible to slow down the degenerative course by staging and earlier detection of CKD. By earlier recognition, supportive treatment (or avoiding further renal insults) can be initiated earlier and life potentially prolonged.

DISCLOSURE

The authors have nothing to disclose.

REFERENCES

1. Schott HC 2nd, Patterson KS, Fitzgerald SD, et al. Chronic renal failure in 99 horses. In: AAEP Annual Convention Proceedings. 1997. Available at: https://www.researchgate.net/profile/Harold_Schott_II/publication/238709884_Chronic_Renal_Failure_in_99_Horses/links/0046352bc7b0d7b01c000000/Chronic-Renal-Failure-in-99-Horses.pdf. Accessed July 18, 2021.
2. O'neill DG, Elliott J, Church DB, et al. Chronic kidney disease in dogs in UK veterinary practices: prevalence, risk factors, and survival. J Vet Intern Med 2013; 27(4):814–21.

3. O'Neill DG, Church DB, McGreevy PD, et al. Longevity and mortality of cats attending primary care veterinary practices in England. J Feline Med Surg 2015;17(2):125–33.

4. Levin A, Stevens PE, Bilous RW, et al. Kidney Disease: Improving Global Outcomes (KDIGO) CKD Work Group. KDIGO 2012 clinical practice guideline for the evaluation and management of chronic kidney disease. Kidney Int supplements 2013;3(1):1–150.

5. Lippi I, Bonelli F, Meucci V, et al. Estimation of glomerular filtration rate by plasma clearance of iohexol in healthy horses of various ages. J Vet Intern Med 2019;33(6):2765–9.

6. Savage VL, Marr CM, Bailey M, et al. Prevalence of acute kidney injury in a population of hospitalized horses. J Vet Intern Med 2019;33(5):2294–301.

7. Laurberg M, van Galen G, Jacobsen S, et al. 13th Annual European College of Equine Internal Medicine Congress. J Vet Intern Med 2021;35(2):1177–93.

8. Schott HC 2nd. Chronic renal failure in horses. Vet Clin North Am Equine Pract 2007;23(3):593–612, vi.

9. Laverty S, Pascoe JR, Ling GV, et al. Urolithiasis in 68 horses. Vet Surg 1992;21(1):56–62.

10. Kisthardt KK, Schumacher J, Finn-Bodner ST, et al. Severe renal hemorrhage caused by pyelonephritis in 7 horses: clinical and ultrasonographic evaluation. Can Vet J 1999;40(8):571–6.

11. Behm RJ, Berg IE. Hematuria caused by renal medullary crest necrosis in a horse. The compendium on continuing education for the practicing veterinarian (USA). 1987. Available at: https://agris.fao.org/agris-search/search.do?recordID=US875386088. Accessed July 18, 2021.

12. Navas de Solis C, Slack J, Boston RC, et al. Hypertensive cardiomyopathy in horses: 5 cases (1995-2011). J Am Vet Med Assoc 2013;243(1):126–30.

13. Frye MA, Johnson JS, Traub-Dargatz JL, et al. Putative uremic encephalopathy in horses: five cases (1978-1998). J Am Vet Med Assoc 2001;218(4):560–6.

14. Kim DM, Lee IH, Song CJ. Uremic encephalopathy: MR imaging findings and clinical correlation. AJNR Am J Neuroradiol 2016;37(9):1604–9.

15. Schott HC 2nd, Esser MM. The sick adult horse: renal clinical pathologic testing and urinalysis. Vet Clin North Am Equine Pract 2020;36(1):121–34.

16. Smith BP, Van Metre DC, Pusterla N. Large animal Internal medicine - E-Book. St. Louis, Missouri: Elsevier Health Sciences; 2019.

17. Hokamp JA, Nabity MB. Renal biomarkers in domestic species. Vet Clin Pathol 2016;45(1):28–56.

18. Finco DR. Measurement of glomerular filtration rate via urinary clearance of inulin and plasma clearance of technetium Tc 99m pentetate and exogenous creatinine in dogs. Am J Vet Res 2005;66(6):1046–55.

19. McKenna M, Pelligand L, Elliott J, et al. Clinical utility of estimation of glomerular filtration rate in dogs. J Vet Intern Med 2020;34(1):195–205.

20. Wilson KE, Wilcke JR, Crisman MV, et al. Comparison of serum iohexol clearance and plasma creatinine clearance in clinically normal horses. Am J Vet Res 2009;70(12):1545–50.

21. Finch NC, Syme HM, Elliott J. Development of an estimated glomerular filtration rate formula in cats. J Vet Intern Med 2018;32(6):1970–6.

22. Manoeuvrier G, Bach-Ngohou K, Batard E, et al. Diagnostic performance of serum blood urea nitrogen to creatinine ratio for distinguishing prerenal from

intrinsic acute kidney injury in the emergency department. BMC Nephrol 2017; 18(1). https://doi.org/10.1186/s12882-017-0591-9.

23. Uchino S, Bellomo R, Goldsmith D. The meaning of the blood urea nitrogen/ creatinine ratio in acute kidney injury. Clin Kidney J 2012;5(2):187–91.

24. Gratwick Z. An updated review: laboratory investigation of equine renal disease. Equine Vet Educ 2020. https://doi.org/10.1111/eve.13373. eve.13373.

25. Topham P. Proteinuric renal disease. Clin Med 2009;9(3):284–7.

26. Martorelli CR, Kogika MM, Chacar FC, et al. Urinary fractional excretion of phosphorus in dogs with spontaneous chronic kidney disease. Vet Sci China 2017; 4(4). https://doi.org/10.3390/vetsci4040067.

27. Remuzzi G, Perico N, Macia M, et al. The role of renin-angiotensin-aldosterone system in the progression of chronic kidney disease. Kidney Int Suppl 2005;(99):S57–65.

28. Chen TK, Knicely DH, Grams ME. Chronic kidney disease diagnosis and management: a review. JAMA 2019;322(13):1294–304.

29. Acierno MJ, Brown S, Coleman AE, et al. ACVIM consensus statement: guidelines for the identification, evaluation, and management of systemic hypertension in dogs and cats. J Vet Intern Med 2018;32(6):1803–22.

30. Olsen E, Pedersen TLS, Robinson R, et al. Accuracy and precision of oscillometric blood pressure in standing conscious horses. J Vet Emerg Crit Care 2016; 26(1):85–92.

31. Heliczer N, Lorello O, Casoni D, et al. Accuracy and precision of noninvasive blood pressure in normo-, hyper-, and hypotensive standing and anesthetized adult horses. J Vet Intern Med 2016;30(3):866–72.

32. Sargent HJ, Elliott J, Jepson RE. The new age of renal biomarkers: does SDMA solve all of our problems? J Small Anim Pract 2021;62(2):71–81.

33. Schott HC 2nd, Gallant LR, Coyne M, et al. Symmetric dimethylarginine and creatinine concentrations in serum of healthy draft horses. J Vet Intern Med 2021;35(2):1147–54.

34. Siwinska N, Zak A, Paslawska U. Detecting acute kidney injury in horses by measuring the concentration of symmetric dimethylarginine in serum. Acta Vet Scand 2021;63(1). https://doi.org/10.1186/s13028-021-00568-0.

35. Siwinska N, Zak A, Slowikowska M, et al. Serum symmetric dimethylarginine concentration in healthy horses and horses with acute kidney injury. BMC Vet Res 2020;16(1). https://doi.org/10.1186/s12917-020-02621-y.

36. Jacobsen S, Berg LC, Tvermose E, et al. Validation of an ELISA for detection of neutrophil gelatinase-associated lipocalin (NGAL) in equine serum. Vet Clin Pathol 2018;47(4):603–7.

37. Uberti B, Eberle DB, Pressler BM, et al. Determination of and correlation between urine protein excretion and urine protein-to-creatinine ratio values during a 24-hour period in healthy horses and ponies. Am J Vet Res 2009;70(12): 1551–6.

38. Bandari J, Fuller TW, Turner Ii RM, et al. Renal biopsy for medical renal disease: indications and contraindications. Can J Urol 2016;23(1):8121–6.

39. Tyner GA, Nolen-Walston RD, Hall T, et al. A Multicenter Retrospective Study of 151 Renal Biopsies in Horses. J Vet Intern Med 2011;25(3):532–9.

40. Eiro M, Katoh T, Watanabe T. Risk factors for bleeding complications in percutaneous renal biopsy. Clin Exp Nephrol 2005;9(1):40–5.

41. Christensen J, Lindequist S, Ulrik Knudsen D, et al. Ultrasound-guided renal biopsy with biopsy gun technique — efficacy and complications. Acta Radiol 1995;36(3):276–9.

42. Kim D, Kim H, Shin G, et al. A randomized, prospective, comparative study of manual and automated renal biopsies. Am J Kidney Dis 1998;32(3):426–31.
43. Walker PD, Cavallo T, Bonsib SM. Ad Hoc Committee on Renal Biopsy Guidelines of the Renal Pathology Society. Practice guidelines for the renal biopsy. Mod Pathol 2004;17(12):1555–63.
44. Scaglione FE, Catalano D, Bestonso R, et al. Comparison between light and electron microscopy in canine and feline renal pathology: a preliminary study. J Microsc 2008;232(3):387–94.
45. Chawla LS, Eggers PW, Star RA, et al. Acute kidney injury and chronic kidney disease as interconnected syndromes. N Engl J Med 2014;371(1):58–66.
46. Chawla LS, Kimmel PL. Acute kidney injury and chronic kidney disease: an integrated clinical syndrome. Kidney Int 2012;82(5):516–24.
47. Ferenbach DA, Bonventre JV. Acute kidney injury and chronic kidney disease: from the laboratory to the clinic. Nephrol Ther 2016;12(Suppl 1):S41–8.
48. Cowgill LD, Polzin DJ, Elliott J, et al. Is progressive chronic kidney disease a slow acute kidney injury? Vet Clin North Am Small Anim Pract 2016;46(6):995–1013.
49. Yerramilli M, Farace G, Quinn J, et al. Kidney disease and the nexus of chronic kidney disease and acute kidney injury: the role of novel biomarkers as early and accurate diagnostics. Vet Clin North Am Small Anim Pract 2016;46(6):961–93.
50. Sato Y, Yanagita M. Immune cells and inflammation in AKI to CKD progression. Am J Physiology-Renal Physiol 2018;315(6):F1501–12.
51. Schnaper HW. The tubulointerstitial pathophysiology of progressive kidney disease. Adv Chronic Kidney Dis 2017;24(2):107–16.
52. Divers TJ, Whitlock RH, Byars TD, et al. Acute renal failure in six horses resulting from haemodynamic causes. Equine Vet J 1987;19(3):178–84.
53. Read WK. Renal medullary crest necrosis associated with phenylbutazone therapy in horses. Vet Pathol 1983;20(6):662–9.
54. de Roij van Zuijdewijn C, van Dorp W, Florquin S, et al. Bisphosphonate nephropathy: a case series and review of the literature. Br J Clin Pharmacol 2021;17. https://doi.org/10.1111/bcp.14780.
55. Toller CS, Charlesworth S, Mihalyo M, et al. Bisphosphonates: AHFS 92:24. J Pain Symptom Manage 2019;57(5):1018–30.
56. Casteel SW. Metal toxicosis in horses. Vet Clin North Am Equine Pract 2001;17(3):517–27.
57. Divers TJ, Timoney JF, Lewis RM, et al. Equine glomerulonephritis and renal failure associated with complexes of group-C streptococcal antigen and IgG antibody. Vet Immunol Immunopathol 1992;32(1–2):93–102.
58. Divers TJ, Byars TD, Shin SJ. Renal dysfunction associated with infection of Leptospira interrogans in a horse. J Am Vet Med Assoc 1992;201(9):1391–2.
59. Divers TJ, Chang Y-F, Irby NL, et al. Leptospirosis: an important infectious disease in North American horses. Equine Vet J 2019;51(3):287–92.
60. Banks KL, KI B, Jb H, et al. Immunologically mediated glomerulitis of horses. I. Pathogenesis in persistent infection by equine infectious anemia virus. Lab Invest 1972;26(6):701–7.
61. Roberts MC, Kelly WR. Renal dysfunction in a case of purpura haemorrhagica in a horse. Vet Rec 1982;110(7):144–6.
62. Divers TJ. Nephrolithiasis and ureterolithiasis in horses and their association with renal disease and failure. Equine Vet J 1989;21(3):161–2.

63. Ehnen SJ, Divers TJ, Gillette D, et al. Obstructive nephrolithiasis and ureteroli-thiasis associated with chronic renal failure in horses: eight cases (1981-1987). J Am Vet Med Assoc 1990;197(2):249–53.
64. Duesterdieck-Zellmer KF. Equine urolithiasis. Vet Clin North Am Equine Pract 2007;23(3):613–629, vi.
65. Saetra T, Breuhaus B, Hildebran A. Unilateral nephrolithiasis with renal rupture in a horse. Equine Vet Education 2018;30(12):635–9.
66. Macbeth BJ. Obstructive urolithiasis, unilateral hydronephrosis, and probable nephrolithiasis in a 12-year-old Clydesdale gelding. Can Vet J 2008;49(3): 287–90.
67. Schott HC II. Recurrent urolithiasis associated with unilateral pyelonephritis in five equids. Proc Am Ass Equine Practnrs 2002;48:136–7. Citeseer.
68. Mair TS, Osborn RS. The crystalline composition of normal equine urine de-posits. Equine Vet J 1990;22(5):364–5.
69. Osborne CA, Albasan H, Lulich JP, et al. Quantitative analysis of 4468 uroliths retrieved from farm animals, exotic species, and wildlife submitted to the Minne-sota Urolith Center: 1981 to 2007. Vet Clin North Am Small Anim Pract 2009; 39(1):65–78.
70. Queau Y. Nutritional Management of Urolithiasis. Vet Clin North Am Small Anim Pract 2019;49(2):175–86.
71. Milligan M, Berent AC. Medical and interventional management of upper urinary tract uroliths. Vet Clin North Am Small Anim Pract 2019;49(2):157–74.
72. Aslani M, Askari AH. Nephrolithiasis in two Arabian horses. Iranian J Vet Sci Technology 2009;1(1):53–7.
73. Frederick J, Freeman DE, MacKay RJ, et al. Removal of ureteral calculi in two geldings via a standing flank approach. J Am Vet Med Assoc 2012;241(9): 1214–20.
74. Rodger LD, Carlson GP, Moran ME, et al. Resolution of a left ureteral stone using electrohydraulic lithotripsy in a thoroughbred colt. J Vet Intern Med 1995;9(4): 280–2.
75. Juzwiak JS, Bain FT, Slone DE, et al. Unilateral nephrectomy for treatment of chronic hematuria due to nephrolithiasis in a colt. Can Vet J 1988;29(11):931–3.
76. Röcken M, Mosel G, Stehle C, et al. Laparoscopy assisted nephrectomy in a standing horse suffering from nephrolithiasis. Pferdeheilkunde Equine Med 2005;21(3):204–10.
77. Frye MA. Pathophysiology, diagnosis, and management of urinary tract infection in horses. Vet Clin North Am Equine Pract 2006;22(2):497–517, x.
78. Van Kampen KR. Sudan grass and sorghum poisoning of horses: a possible lathyrogenic disease. J Am Vet Med Assoc 1970;156(5):629–30.
79. Abbasi MA, Chertow GM, Hall YN. End-stage renal disease. BMJ Clin Evid 2010;2010. Available at: https://www.ncbi.nlm.nih.gov/pubmed/21418665.
80. Betjes MGH. Immune cell dysfunction and inflammation in end-stage renal dis-ease. Nat Rev Nephrol 2013;9(5):255–65.
81. Siudak K, Stallenberger L, Herden C, et al. Renal neoplasia in horses – a retro-spective study. Tierärztliche Praxis Ausgabe G: Großtiere/Nutztiere 2017;45(05): 290–5.
82. Wise LN, Bryan JN, Sellon DC, et al. A retrospective analysis of renal carcinoma in the horse. J Vet Intern Med 2009;23(4):913–8.
83. Romero A, Rodgerson DH, Fontaine GL. Hand-assisted laparoscopic removal of a nephroblastoma in a horse. Can Vet J 2010;51(6):637–9.

84. Matsuda K, Kousaka Y, Nagamine N, et al. Papillary renal adenoma of distal nephron differentiation in a horse. J Vet Med Sci 2007;69(7):763–5.

85. Andrews FM, Rosol TJ, Kohn CW, et al. Bilateral renal hypoplasia in four young horses. J Am Vet Med Assoc 1986;189(2):209–12.

86. Gough SL, Fraser BSL, Rendle DI, et al. Renal dysplasia, ectopic ureter, septic ureterectasia and cryptorchidism in an 11-month-old Cob colt presenting with ascending pyoureter and pyocystis. Equine Vet Educ 2020. https://doi.org/10.1111/eve.13296. eve.13296.

87. Wooldridge AA, Seahorn TL, Williams J, et al. Chronic renal failure associated with nephrolithiasis, ureterolithiasis, and renal dysplasia in a 2-year-old quarter horse gelding. Vet Radiol Ultrasound 1999;40(4):361–4.

88. Bertone JJ, Traub-Dargatz JL, Fettman MJ, et al. Monitoring the progression of renal failure in a horse with polycystic kidney disease: use of the reciprocal of serum creatinine concentration and sodium sulfanilate clearance half-time. J Am Vet Med Assoc 1987;191(5):565–8.

89. Aguilera-Tejero E, Estepa JC, López I, et al. Polycystic kidneys as a cause of chronic renal failure and secondary hypoparathyroidism in a horse. Equine Vet J 2000;32(2):167–9.

90. Saam D. Urethrolithiasis and nephrolithiasis in a horse. Can Vet J 2001;42(11):880–3.

91. Birkmann K, Trump M, Dettwiler M, et al. Severe polyuria and polydipsia as major clinical signs in a horse with unilateral renal adenocarcinoma. Equine Vet Education 2016;28(12):675–80.

92. Peters M, Grafen J, Kuhnen C, et al. Malignant glomus tumour (glomangiosarcoma) with additional neuroendocrine differentiation in a horse. J Comp Pathol 2016;154(4):309–13.

93. Hughes K, Scott VHL, Blanck M, et al. Equine renal hemangiosarcoma: clinical presentation, pathologic features, and pSTAT3 expression. J Vet Diagn Invest 2018;30(2):268–74.

94. Vaden SL, Elliott J. Management of proteinuria in dogs and cats with chronic kidney disease. Vet Clin North Am Small Anim Pract 2016;46(6):1115–30.

95. Vandendriessche VL, Dufourni A, Loon G, et al. Successful nutritional management of a 21-year-old quarter horse gelding with acute renal failure. Vet Rec Case Rep 2016;4(1):e000309.

96. Saran R, Novak JE, Desai A, et al. Impact of vitamin E on plasma asymmetric dimethylarginine (ADMA) in chronic kidney disease (CKD): a pilot study. Nephrol Dial Transpl 2003;18(11):2415–20.

97. Signorini L, Granata S, Lupo A, et al. Naturally occurring compounds: new potential weapons against oxidative stress in chronic kidney disease. Int J Mol Sci 2017;18(7). https://doi.org/10.3390/ijms18071481.

98. Heiwe S, Jacobson SH. Exercise training in adults with CKD: a systematic review and meta-analysis. Am J Kidney Dis 2014;64(3):383–93.

99. Pei G, Tang Y, Tan L, et al. Aerobic exercise in adults with chronic kidney disease (CKD): a meta-analysis. Int Urol Nephrol 2019;51(10):1787–95.

100. Wong DM, Ruby RE, Eatroff A, et al. Use of renal replacement therapy in a neonatal foal with postresuscitation acute renal failure. J Vet Intern Med 2017;31(2):593–7.

101. Peek SF. Peritoneal dialysis and acute renal failure: a new treatment for an old disease? Equine Vet Educ 2008;20(5):265–6.

102. Gallatin LL, Couëtil LL, Ash SR. Use of continuous-flow peritoneal dialysis for the treatment of acute renal failure in an adult horse. J Am Vet Med Assoc 2005; 226(5):756–9, 732.
103. Han JH, McKenzie HC III. Intermittent peritoneal dialysis for the treatment of acute renal failure in two horses. Equine Vet Educ 2008;20(5):256–64.
104. Ruiz-Ortega M, Rayego-Mateos S, Lamas S, et al. Targeting the progression of chronic kidney disease. Nat Rev Nephrol 2020;16(5):269–88.
105. Schmitz, David G. Toxins Affecting the Urinary System. The Veterinary Clinics of North America. Equine Practice 2007;23(3):677–770.

Urinary Tract Disorders of Foals

SallyAnne L. DeNotta, DVM, PhD

KEYWORDS

- Urinary • Foal • Uroperitoneum • Urachus • Bladder • Neonate • Urinalysis • Renal

KEY POINTS

- Equine neonates produce hyposthenuric urine, and serial measurement of urine specific gravity is an inexpensive and noninvasive method for monitoring hydration status in sick foals.
- Elevated serum creatinine concentrations (occasionally >15 mg/dL) in newborn foals reflect abnormal placental circulation in utero and can be observed in foals with hypoxic-ischemic injury or foals born to mares with placental insufficiency. This "spurious hypercreatininemia" syndrome is associated with normal renal function, serum electrolytes, and urinalysis, and serum creatinine concentrations generally decline to normal concentrations within the first 1 to 3 days of life.
- Uroperitoneum can be diagnosed via abdominal ultrasound and confirmed by comparing peritoneal fluid and serum creatinine concentrations. *It is important to stabilize the patient and address hyperkalemia, if present, before attempting surgical intervention.*
- Ultrasound examination of the urinary bladder, kidneys, umbilical vein, umbilical arteries, and urachal remnants can assist in the diagnosis of common neonatal urinary disorders.

INTRODUCTION

Urinary disease in the neonatal period can occur with primary congenital renal defects or as a secondary consequence of birth trauma, ischemic injury, nephrotoxic medications, or systemic illness. This article reviews the clinical evaluation of the urinary system in foals and highlights diagnostic and therapeutic features of the most commonly encountered urinary disorders of the equine neonatal patient.

CLINICAL EVALUATION OF THE URINARY SYSTEM IN FOALS

Evaluation of the newborn foal with suspected urinary disease should begin with careful physical examination. The average time to first urination is 6 hours in colts and up to 11 hours in fillies.[1] In male foals, the penis is not easily extracted from the prepuce

Department of Large Animal Clinical Sciences, College of Veterinary Medicine, University of Florida, PO Box 10036, Gainesville, FL 32610, USA
E-mail address: s.denotta@ufl.edu

Vet Clin Equine 38 (2022) 47–56
https://doi.org/10.1016/j.cveq.2021.11.004
0749-0739/22/© 2021 Elsevier Inc. All rights reserved.

without sedation, and many normal colts do not exteriorize the penis to urinate for the first few days of life. Because normal suckling foals consume large volumes of milk (up to 25% body weight per day), they urinate frequently and produce large volumes of low specific gravity urine, often up to 148 mL/kg per day in healthy foals.[2] Although frequent urination is a normal observation, unproductive straining, frequent "tail flagging," and/or constant urine dribbling are abnormal behaviors that should alert clinicians to an underlying problem. Dysuria or stranguria can be observed in foals with uroperitoneum, urachitis, patent urachus, cystitis, cystic blood clots secondary to internal umbilical hemorrhage, or from neonatal encephalopathy. Subcutaneous edema in the inguinal and axially regions may be observed in oliguric foals. Focal swelling surrounding the umbilical stump can result from subcutaneous urine accumulation in foals with urachal tears. The umbilicus should be palpated for enlargement, herniation, and discharge. A wet umbilical stump or overt umbilical urine dribbling is indicative of a patent urachus, a commonly observed condition in sick or weak foals. Obvious incontinence (constant urine dribbling) or evidence of urine scalding is suggestive of ectopic ureters, whereas intermittent straining to urinate is commonly observed in foals with urethritis and/or cystitis (often secondary to urinary catheterization) and occasionally in colts with urethral impingement secondary to meconium impaction. Urine that is opaque or "cheeselike" in appearance is a clinical sign of systemic candidiasis and can occur in foals treated with long-term antimicrobial therapy. In these cases, the presence of funguria may be confirmed with urinalysis, and if treatment is required, oral fluconazole is the treatment of choice.[3]

Serial measurement of urine specific gravity (USG) is an inexpensive and noninvasive method for monitoring hydration status in sick foals. Neonatal urine may be initially dilute or concentrated (USG up 1.040 during first day of life) but should rapidly become hyposthenuric (USG <1.008) within 24 hours of age in foals that are nursing appropriately. Compared with that of adult horses, foal urine is more acidic (pH 5.5–8.0) and has increased protein (2–3+ proteinuria on urine reagent strips) for the first 36 hours of life because of colostral antibody absorption and subsequent renal protein excretion.[4] Neonatal kidneys are fully functional at birth, with newborn foals demonstrating glomerular filtration rates and electrolyte fractional excretion profiles similar to that of adult horses.[4–6]

Azotemia is defined as elevations in serum creatinine (Cr) and/or serum urea nitrogen (BUN) and can be observed in neonatal foals as an indicator of prerenal hypoperfusion, acute intrinsic kidney disease or failure, congenital renal disorders, and uroperitoneum. Both Cr and BUN concentrations are variable within the first 24 hours of life, dropping to less than 1.0 mg/dL and less than 10 mg/dL by 1 to 2 weeks of age, respectively.[7–9] These low values reflect diuresis secondary to the large fluid volume consumed as milk and persist as long as the foal maintains an all-milk diet.[2] Elevated serum Cr concentrations (occasionally >15 mg/dL) in newborn foals most commonly reflect abnormal placental circulation in utero and can be observed in foals with hypoxic-ischemic injury or foals born to mares with placental insufficiency.[10] This "spurious hypercreatininemia" syndrome is associated with normal renal function, serum electrolytes and urinalysis, and serum Cr concentrations generally decline to normal concentrations within the first 1 to 3 days of life. Serum symmetric dimethylarginine (SDMA), a renally excreted byproduct of protein catabolism, has garnered recent attention as a possible biomarker for early detection of kidney dysfunction in horses. A recent study evaluating adult horses and foals as young as 2 months of age found that healthy foals had higher SDMA concentrations (median 1.5 μmol/L) when compared with healthy adult horses (median 0.54 μmol/L)[11]; however, there are no published reports of SDMA concentrations in neonatal foals at the time of this review.

Sick foals with adequate renal function and prerenal azotemia secondary to dehydration and/or renal hypoperfusion typically display normal serum electrolyte concentrations, USG $\geq$1.025, and urine osmolality $\geq$500 mOsm/kg. In contrast, foals with intrinsic renal disease lose the ability to concentrate or dilute urine, often presenting with isosthenuric urine (USG 1.009–1.014), urine osmolality less than 300 mOsm/Kg, and alternations in serum electrolyte concentrations and acid base status, including hyponatremia, hypochloremia, hyperkalemia, and metabolic acidosis.[9] Intrinsic renal disease is further supported by evidence of tubular damage, including proteinuria, microscopic hematuria, glucosuria, and increased fractional excretions of sodium and chloride.

In addition to physical examination and clinicopathologic assessment, ultrasonography is an important component of the diagnostic workup of foals with urinary disease. Transabdominal sonography of neonatal urinary and umbilical structures can be achieved using linear, sector, or rectal ultrasound probes with the foal standing or in lateral recumbency. Confirmation of 2 kidneys of normal shape and size (approximately 5 $\times$ 10 cm for a 50-kg foal)[12] is followed by evaluation of the urinary bladder, internal umbilical remnant structures (umbilical vein, umbilical arteries, urachus), and external umbilical stump. Detailed descriptions of umbilical sonographic examination technique is described elsewhere.[13] Briefly, the external umbilical stump is scanned for evidence of sepsis up to the point where it crossed the body wall, and the internal umbilical vein is followed cranially as it courses to the liver. Intraluminal thrombi are normal. Caudal to the umbilical stump, the paired umbilical arteries and the urachus are imaged together as they course toward the bladder. The paired umbilical arteries diverge to course along the lateral aspect of the bladder and are often asymmetrical in size. A recent study of healthy Standardbred foals reported a median umbilical vein diameter of 0.83 cm, median umbilical artery diameter of 0.61 cm, and median urachal diameter of 1.07 cm. All structures were largest at 24 hours of age and rapidly regressed over the first few weeks of life.[14] Renal pelvises may appear symmetrically dilated in foals receiving intravenous fluid therapy.[9] The urinary bladder should be assessed for size, and a urinary catheter passed if the bladder diameter is found to be >10 cm. Small bladder size may be indicative of recent voiding or oliguria, whereas large, turgid bladders may be observed in recumbent or maladjusted foals with poor detrusor tone or bladder sphincter dyssynergia (this syndrome is sometimes referred to as "Dummy foal bladder" and can precede bladder rupture in hospitalized foals). Hypoechoic free peritoneal fluid is a hallmark finding in foals with uroperitoneum, and careful examination of the urachus and urinary bladder may reveal the site of rupture. Bladders with small leaks may maintain intraluminal urine and a rounded appearance on ultrasound.

ACUTE KIDNEY INJURY AND ACUTE RENAL FAILURE

Intrinsic renal disease and acute renal failure can develop as a consequence of hypoxic-ischemic injury (vasomotor nephropathy), septicemia, infection with *Leptospirosis interrogans*, or toxicity secondary to nephrotoxic medications. Vasomotor nephropathy results from insufficient blood flow and/or disturbances in intrarenal vasoconstrictor-vasodilator forces. Septic, hypotensive, and hypovolemic foals, especially those with diarrhea or respiratory failure, are at considerable risk of developing vasomotor nephropathy, and both urine output and serum Cr levels should be monitored closely in all hospitalized neonates. Neonatal renal injury is often multifactorial, as sick or compromised foals are routinely treated with aminoglycoside antimicrobials and nonsteroidal anti-inflammatory drugs, both of which have the potential to induce or exacerbate renal injury. Tetracyclines are also nephrotoxic and often administered in high doses to neonates for the treatment of contracted tendons. Nephrotoxic drugs should be used only in euvolemic foals that are producing an adequate amount of urine, and only with careful patient monitoring in any neonatal patient. Acute kidney failure has also been reported in septicemic foals with fibrin thromboemboli and renal infarction secondary to intravascular coagulation activation.[15]

Foals with intrinsic renal failure have similar biochemical alternations to adult horses, with elevations in serum Cr and BUN, as well as serum electrolyte derangements, including hyponatremia, hypochloremia, and hyperkalemia. Urinalysis reveals isosthenuric urine along with indicators of tubular injury, including proteinuria, microscopic hematuria, glucosuria, and increased fractional excretion of sodium and chloride. Urine sediment examination may reveal hyaline or granular casts, further supporting damage to the renal tubules. Foals with renal failure secondary to *Leptospirosis* spp infection may have additional clinical signs of systemic sepsis, including fever and abnormal leukograms.[16–18]

Treatment of foals with acute kidney injury or acute renal failure is focused on removing nephrotoxic medications, correcting electrolyte derangements, treating underlying infection, and maintaining renal blood flow and urine output. Whenever possible, urine output should be quantified to identify oliguric foals (<0.5–1.0 mL/kg per hour urine output), as these patients carry a more guarded prognosis and may require pharmacologic intervention to bolster urine production and prevent the development of anuric renal failure. Indwelling bladder catheters with urine collection systems can be used to measure "ins" and "outs," although these carry an increased risk of iatrogenic ascending urinary tract infection and can be logistically difficult to maintain in freely ambulating foals. After the correction of intravascular volume deficits, Isotonic crystalloids should be administered at approximately 1.0 to 2.0 mL/kg per hour and patients monitored for changes in urine production, body weight or development of edema.[9] Foals that remain oliguric in the face of intravenous fluid therapy may benefit from diuretic therapy. Furosemide may be administered at 1 to 3 mg/kg intravenously every 2 hours or as a constant rate infusion (CRI) at 0.12 mg/kg per hour intravenously. Furosemide is a loop diuretic, and foals receiving repeated treatment and/or constant infusion should be monitored closely for the development of hypokalemia. Vasopressor agents, including dopamine, norepinephrine, and dobutamine, can be used as constant rate infusions to increase renal perfusion,[19] but the need for intensive monitoring of common side effects, including hypertension and cardiac arrythmias, limit their use outside of hospital settings.

PATENT URACHUS

The urachus is the structure through which fetal urine passes into the allantoic cavity in utero. Failure of the urachus to close at birth, or reestablishment of patency in the neonatal period, leads to urine leakage from the umbilical stump. Leaked urine volume can range from a persistently moist umbilicus to a full urine stream during micturition. Local sepsis, including omphalitis and omphalophlebitis, are common risk factors for the development of a patent urachus, but may also occur as secondary consequences of persistent urine leakage and contamination.[20,21] Weak, sick, or otherwise compromised foals may also develop a patent urachus during hospitalization as a result of recumbency and abnormal voiding behavior. Foals found to be leaking urine from the umbilicus should be evaluated via transabdominal ultrasound for evidence of infected internal umbilical remnants, including the urachus, umbilical arteries, and umbilical vein. Many uncomplicated cases of patent urachus will resolve with supportive care, routine umbilical disinfection, and systemic antimicrobial therapy if needed. Empiric treatment with broad-spectrum antimicrobials eliminated and concentrated in the urine may includes cephalosporins, potentiated sulfonamides, aminoglycosides, and/or penicillins. Umbilical dips aimed at reducing bacterial populations on the umbilicus can be performed multiple times a day using 0.5% chlorhexidine or dilute betadine solutions. Surgical resection of the umbilical remnants is often recommended for foals with obviously septic umbilical structures, and/or those who fail to respond to several days of medical management. Surgical management is associated with overall favorable long-term outcomes.[20,21] For foals without evidence of umbilical sepsis, chemical cautery of the umbilical stump can be attempted by carefully using silver nitrate applicators or swabs dipped in 7% iodine solution. Care should be taken to not allow any caustic cautery agents to contact the body wall, as additional tissue irritation may further predispose to infection.

UROPERITONEUM

Uroperitoneum most commonly occurs in colts that sustain dorsal bladder wall tears while passing through the birth canal, although the condition is also observed in fillies. Clinical signs may take 1 to 3 days to develop and include abdominal distension, colic, lethargy, anorexia, and straining to urinate.[22,23] Foals with bladder leaks can often still urinate, and observing a normal urine stream does not rule out a uroabdomen. Bladder ruptures may also occur in several-days-old sick foals with generalized weakness and poor detrusor tone. This syndrome, sometimes referred to as "dummy foal bladder," appears to be a component of neonatal maladjustment syndrome and is more common in recumbent foals receiving fluid therapy. Extreme caution should be taken when repositioning recumbent foals or assisting weak foals to stand, as pressure on the abdomen may lead to bladder rupture in foals with incomplete bladder emptying. Maladjusted foals may also present with bladder sphincter dyssynergia, a condition characterized by uncoordinated detrusor contraction against a contracted external urethral sphincter. A retrospective study of uroperitoneum in hospitalized foals found no gender predilection, and positive sepsis scores in approximately half of affected foals.[22] Thus, clinicians are encouraged to monitor urine output vigilantly in sick compromised foals and use abdominal ultrasound to monitor for bladder distention and inadequate voiding. In foals suspected of having inadequate detrusor function, placement of an indwelling urinary catheter for a few days can prevent both bladder rupture and additional detrusor stretch injury (**Fig. 1**). In most foals with "dummy foal bladder," detrusor function and micturition behavior generally normalize within 1 to 5 days. Foals that strain in response to urethral irritation from indwelling catheters often respond favorably to treatment with phenazopyridine HCl, which is excreted into the urine, where it exerts local analgesic effects on the urinary tract mucosa. Phenazopyridine HCl is administered at a dose of 4 mg/kg orally every 8 to 12 hours and results in bright-orange–stained urine.

Uroperitoneum may also be observed in foals with urachal tears, a condition that often occurs as a consequence of septic omphalitis and subsequent focal tissue necrosis. If the urachal defect is adjacent or external to the body wall, urine accumulation within the abdominal fascia and subcutaneous tissues leads to marked swelling and focal edema around the umbilicus (**Fig. 2**). Careful ultrasound examination of internal umbilical structures may reveal urachal defects and local fluid dissection into adjacent tissues (**Fig. 3**). Although surgical umbilical resection is the most commonly recommended therapy for urachal tears, medical management may also be effective for foals without a surgical option. Indwelling bladder catheters can be used to facilitate

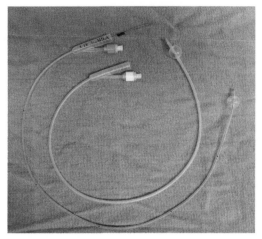

Fig. 1. 8F and 10F Foley silicone catheters (55–60 cm in length) appropriate for bladder catheterization in fillies and colts. Removable wire stylets provide stiffness and facilitate catheter passage. Filling the balloon with saline instead of air prevents deflation and inadvertent removal.

urine passage and allow the urachal tissue defect to close. Catheters may be left in place for several days; however, multidrug-resistant cystitis is a common sequela, and prophylactic therapy with broad-spectrum, renally excreted antimicrobials is indicated. Rarely, uroperitoneum may occur secondary to unilateral or bilateral ureteral defects. If the defect is located in the proximal ureter near the kidney, urine may accumulate in the retroperitoneal space. Both intravenous pyelography and CT urography can help aid in the diagnosis of ureteral rupture, and successful surgical correction has been described.[24]

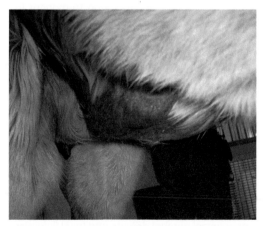

Fig. 2. A 3-day-old colt with a urachal tear leading to urine accumulation in the abdominal fascia and subcutaneous tissues. Note marked swelling and edema surrounding the umbilicus. This foal underwent surgical resection of the umbilical remnants and was treated postoperatively with broad-spectrum antimicrobials.

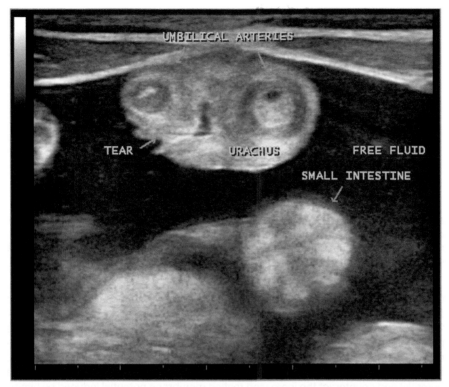

Fig. 3. Transabdominal ultrasound image of the internal umbilical structures just caudal to the umbilical stump in a 2-day-old foal presenting for uroabdomen. A tear can be seen in the urachus as well as hypoechoic free peritoneal fluid later confirmed to be urine.

In all cases of uroperitoneum, abdominal ultrasound provides rapid confirmation of hypoechoic free peritoneal fluid (**Fig. 4**). Although large defects will result in copious volumes of free fluid and a flaccid, empty bladder, bladders with small leaks may maintain intraluminal urine and a rounded appearance on ultrasound. The diagnosis can be confirmed by performing abdominocentesis and comparing serum and perito-neal fluid Cr concentrations. Although urine urea rapidly diffuses across membranes and out of the abdomen, Cr is a comparatively larger molecule and is essentially trapped within the peritoneal space, and peritoneal fluid:serum Cr ratios ≥ 2 are diagnostic for urine within the peritoneal space.[25] Classic serum electrolyte derangements in foals with uroperitoneum reflect an equilibration between plasma and the urine contained within the abdominal cavity and include hyperkalemia, hyponatremia, and hypochloremia. These clinical pathologic trends, however, are not always present and may occur less commonly in hospitalized foals receiving fluid therapy.[22,23]

Treatment for uroperitoneum generally involves stabilization of the patient followed by surgical repair of the bladder defect and resection of the umbilical remnants. It is of great importance to note that *bladder ruptures are not surgical emergencies*, and sta-bilization of the patient via controlled abdominal drainage and therapy directed at cor-recting hyperkalemia are critical for ensuring the foal is a safe anesthetic candidate. Controlled abdominal drainage can be performed using a teat canula or 16F trocar chest tube, with the latter having less chance of occlusion with omentum or mesen-tery. Peritoneal urine should be drained with concurrent administration of intravenous

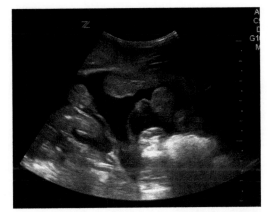

Fig. 4. Hypoechoic free peritoneal fluid identified on transabdominal ultrasound in a 4-day-old Standardbred colt. Peritoneal fluid:serum Cr ratio greater than 2 confirmed the diagnosis of uroperitoneum, and the foal underwent abdominal exploratory surgery, where a defect in the dorsal bladder wall was identified and repaired.

0.9% NaCl to prevent rapid fluid shifts and subsequent hypotension. Hyperkalemic foals should receive supplementation with 5% to 10% dextrose (replace 100–200 mL per liter 0.9% NaCl with 50% dextrose) to stimulate insulin release and drive potassium intracellularly via cell membrane Na/K/ATPase pumps. Additional supplementation with 23% calcium borogluconate solution (50 mL can be added to a 1-L bag of 0.9% NaCl and 5%–10% dextrose solution) helps to raise threshold membrane potential and counteract the increased resting membrane potential induced by hyperkalemia.[26] Serum potassium concentrations should be rechecked every hour, and foals should not be taken to surgery until concentrations ≤5.5 mEq/L are achieved.

HYDROURETER SYNDROME

A poorly described syndrome of unilateral or bilateral hydroureter occurs in neonatal foals and is associated with severe hyponatremia. Foals typically present between 3 and 7 days of age for signs of encephalopathy, blindness, and seizures secondary to sodium concentrations often lower than 110 mEq/L.[25] Affected foals may respond favorably to temporary bladder and ureter catheterization, whereas surgical transposition of the ureteral opening into the bladder may be an effective treatment option if a ureteral flap is identified as the cause of obstruction.

CONGENITAL URINARY DISORDERS

Congenital renal anomalies include renal agenesis and aplasia, hypoplasia, hydronephrosis, and polycystic kidneys.[27,28] There are no known breed or sex predilection. If the anomaly is unilateral or if sufficient numbers of functioning nephrons are present, these anomalies may be identified as incidental findings during abdominal ultrasound examination for complaints unrelated to renal disease. Some foals will ultimately progress to renal failure, whereas others may develop into adulthood without ever developing azotemia or clinical signs of renal disease.[27]

Ectopic ureters are rare in the horse but can occur unilaterally or bilaterally and are more commonly observed in fillies than colts.[29] Urinary incontinence since birth and urine scalding are the most common presenting complaints. Diagnosis can be achieved via antegrade or retrograde ureterography, endoscopic visualization of ectopic ureteral openings within the vagina, and/or computed tomography. Uretero-vesicular anastomosis is an effective surgical method of correction for unilateral or bilateral ectopic ureters and preserves renal function on the affected side. Unilateral nephrectomy is indicated if ipsilateral pyelonephritis or congenital renal dysplasia is present.[29]

DISCLOSURE

The author has nothing to disclose.

REFERENCES

1. Knottenbelt DC. Perinatal review. In: Knottenbelt N, Holdstock NB, Madigan JE, editors. Equine neonatology medicine and surgery. London (UK): WB Saunders; 2004. p. 1–27.
2. Martin RG, McMeniman NP, Dowsett KF. Milk and water intakes of foals sucking grazing mares. Equine Vet J 1992;24:295–9.
3. Reilly LK, Palmer JE. Systemic candidiasis in four foals. J Am Vet Med Assoc 1994;205(3):464–6.
4. Edwards DJ, Brownlow MA, Hutchins DR. Indices of renal function: values in eight normal foals from birth to 56 days. Aust Vet J 1990;67:251–4.
5. Brewer BD, Clement SF, Lotz WS, et al. Renal clearance, urinary excretion of endogenous substances, and urinary diagnostic indices in healthy neonatal foals. J Vet Int Med 1991;5:28–33.
6. Holdstock NB, Ousey JC, Rossdale PD. Glomerular filtration rate, effective renal plasma flow, blood pressure and pulse rate in the equine neonate during the first 10 days post partum. Equine Vet J 1998;30:335–43.
7. Barton MH, Hart KA. Clinical pathology in the foal. Vet Clin North Am Equine Pract 2020;36(1):73–85.
8. Bauer JE. Normal blood chemistry. In: Koterba A, Drummond W, Kosch P, editors. Equine clinical neonatology. Philadelphia (PA): Lea and Febiger; 1990. p. 602–14.
9. Schott HC. Review of azotemia in foals. In: Proceedings of the Annual Convention of the AAEP, Nov 22, 2011, San Antonio, TX; 328–34.
10. Chaney KP, Holcombe SJ, Schott HC, et al. Spurious hypercreatininemia: 28 neonatal foals (2000–2008). J Vet Emerg Crit Care 2010;20:244–9.
11. Siwinska N, Zak A, Slowikowska M, et al. Serum symmetric dimethylarginine concentration in healthy horses and horses with acute kidney injury. BMC Vet Res 2020;16:396.
12. Hoffmann KL, Wood AK, McCarthy PH. Ultrasonography of the equine neonatal kidney. Equine Vet J 2000;32:109–13.
13. Franklin RP, Ferrell EA. How to perform umbilical sonograms in the neonate. In: Proceedings of the Annual Convention of the AAEP, Dec 08, 2002, Orlando, FL; 261–65.
14. McCoy AM, Lopp CT, Kooy S, et al. Normal regression of the internal umbilical remnant structures in standardbred foals. Equine Vet J 2020;52:876–83.
15. Cotovio M, Monreal L, Armengou L, et al. Fibrin deposits and organ failure in newborn foals with severe septicemia. J Vet Intern Med 2008;22:1403–10.
16. Fouche N, Graubner C, Lanz S, et al. Acute kidney injury due to Leptospirosis in-terrogans in 4 foals and use of renal replacement therapy with intermittent hemo-diafiltration in 1 foal. J Vet Intern Med 2020;34:1007–12.

17. Frazer ML. Acute renal failure from leptospirosis in a foal. Aust Vet J 1999;77: 499–500.
18. Frellstedt L, Slovis NM. Acute renal disease from Leptospira interrogans in three yearlings from the same farm. Equine Vet Educ 2009;21:478–84.
19. Hollis AR, Ousey JC, Palmer L, et al. Effects of norepinephrine and a combined norepinephrine and dobutamine infusion on systemic hemodynamics and indices of renal function in normotensive neonatal thoroughbred foals. J Vet Int Med 2006;20:1437–42.
20. Adams SB, Fessler JF. Umbilical remnant infections in foals: 16 cases (1975-1985). J Am Vet Med Assoc 1987;190(3):316–8.
21. Oreff GL, Tatz AJ, Dahan R, et al. Surgical management and long-term outcome of umbilical infection in 65 foals (2010-2015). Vet Surg 2017;46(7):962–70.
22. Kablack KA, Embertson RM, Bernard WV, et al. Uroperitoneum in the hospitalized equine neonate: retrospective study of 31 cases, 1988-1997. Equine Vet J 2010; 32:505–8.
23. Dunkel D, Palmer JE, Olsen KN, et al. Uroperitoneum in 32 foals: influence of intravenous fluid therapy, infection, and sepsis. J Vet Intern Med 2008;19:889–93.
24. Divers TJ, Byars TD, Spirito M. Correction of bilateral ureteral defects in a foal. J Am Vet Med Assoc 1988;192(3):384–6.
25. Magdesian KG. Neonatology. In: Divers TD, Orsini JA, editors. Equine emergency manual. St. Louis (MO): Elsevier; 2014. p. 528–64.
26. Jesty SA. Cardiovascular system. In: Divers TD, Orsini JA, editors. Equine emergency manual. St. Louis (MO): Elsevier; 2014. p. 125–56.
27. Chaney KP. Congenital anomalies of the equine urinary tract. Vet Clin N Am Equine Pract 2007;23:691–6.
28. Gilday RA, Wojnarowicz C, Tryon KA, et al. Bilateral renal dysplasia, hydronephrosis, and hydroureter in a septic neonatal foal. Can Vet J 2015;56:257–60.
29. Pringle JK, Ducharme NG, Baird JD. Ectopic ureter in the horse: three cases and a review of the literature. Can Vet J 1990;31:26–30.

Discolored Urine in Horses and Foals

Barbara Delvescovo, DVM, MRCVS, ACVIM

KEYWORDS

- Discolored urine • Hematuria • Myoglobinuria • Hemoglobinuria

KEY POINTS

- Discolored urine is a common clinical complaint in equine practice.
- It can be difficult to distinguish between hemoglobinuria, myoglobinuria, and sometimes hematuria based on the color of the voided urine alone. Urinary dipsticks also do not distinguish between them.
- Clinical history and examination in addition to a complete urinalysis, hematology, and serum biochemistry will almost always allow determination of pigment causing urine discoloration.
- Bilirubin, methemoglobin, and drug pigments in the urine are less common causes of discolored urine.
- If hematuria is the cause of the discolored urine, ancillary procedures are often required to determine the origin of the hemorrhage.

INTRODUCTION

Normal equine urine can range from a pale-yellow color to a tan color depending on individual variation and concentration. The color is primarily associated with renal excretion of urochrome, a product of the degradation of hemoglobin. Because of the high amount of mucous and calcium carbonate crystals that equine urine physiologically contains, normal appearance can also vary in terms of turbidity, going from transparent to turbid. Equine urine can sometimes stain a brown-red color on bedding or snow. This phenomenon is due to prolonged storage or air exposure and oxidation of plant metabolites (pyrocatechines) and happens right after urine voiding. Abnormal urine color can instead occur because of the presence of blood, pigments, or contaminants. Urinalysis and cytology are important tests aiding in the diagnosis of the discolored urine.

In cases of red discoloration, the reagent strips used for urinalysis indicate a positive result for "blood" when the heme group (porphyrin ring and iron) reacts with peroxidase substrate in the pad. They can reveal heme within the erythrocytes (hematuria), from free hemoglobin (hemoglobinuria) or myoglobin in the urine without being able to

Large Animal Medicine, Cornell University, 930 Campus Road, Ithaca, NY 14850, USA
E-mail address: bd382@cornell.edu

Vet Clin Equine 38 (2022) 57–71
https://doi.org/10.1016/j.cveq.2021.11.005
vetequine.theclinics.com

discriminate among the 3 different sources of discoloration. Differentiation can be achieved with centrifugation and sediment examination. In cases of hematuria, after centrifugation, the red blood cells (RBCs) will deposit and be recognizable upon microscopic evaluation. However, in cases of very diluted urine (specific gravity <1.006), alkaline pH (pH > 8), or delayed analysis, RBCs may not be visible because of possible lysis. In these cases, ghost cells (lysed RBCs that have lost their hemoglobin) may instead be detected. When hemoglobinuria or myoglobinuria is present, the urine does not clear with centrifugation. Myoglobin can be differentiated from hemoglobin through ammonium sulfate precipitation, electrophoresis, or spectroscopy. However, there is usually no need for these additional diagnostics, as clinical findings and biochemical results will help differentiate myoglobinuria from hemoglobinuria. In cases of hemoglobinuria, the serum of the animal will be pink discolored, owing to intravascular hemolysis; patients with myoglobinuria will instead present with clinical signs of myopathy together with severely increased muscle enzymes. False positive heme results on the strips are reported and are usually due to microbial peroxidase activity from bacteria (in cases of urinary tract infections [UTIs]) or strong oxidizing agents, such as hypochlorite (bleach) or povidone-iodine, if the specimen is contaminated.

Urine discoloration with a negative strip result could suggest plant-derived pigments or drug-related discoloration. False negative results are rare. Vitamin C administration has been reported to give false negatives on a blood strip.[1] The collection method of urine should be considered when analyzing samples, as it might influence the interpretation of the results. For example, trauma secondary to catheterization can cause RBCs in the sample, which when present in high numbers, might even cause discoloration. When urine is obtained free catch, the presence of pigment should not be altered; however, several white cells or bacteria might be present because of urine contamination from the genital flora.

Bilirubin positivity on reagent strips can be diagnostic for cholestasis in horses because elevations in conjugated bilirubin will cause bilirubinuria. Only conjugated bilirubin passes freely into urine, because of its water solubility. This might spill into urine before it is even increased in blood. Unconjugated bilirubin is bound to albumin and other carrier proteins and may appear in the urine if proteinuria is present. False positive bilirubin reactions can commonly occur.

DISCUSSION
Hematuria

Normal urine can contain less than 5 RBCs per high-powered field. An increase above this threshold indicates hematuria.[2] Hematuria can be macroscopic, if detectable grossly, or microscopic if not.

As previously mentioned, the presence of red discolored urine (**Fig. 1**) suggests 3 possible pathologic processes: presence of RBCs (hematuria), hemoglobin (hemoglobinuria), or myoglobin (myoglobinuria). Drug metabolites could also give orange-red discoloration. The most commonly reported drug color reactions are due to rifampicin and phenazopyridine's metabolites.

During the diagnostic process, myoglobinuria and hemoglobinuria can be ruled out based on clinical findings and serum biochemistry. In the most severe cases, hematuria is obvious due to voiding of blood clots. Contamination of urine with blood can occur at the level of the kidneys, ureters, bladder, urethra, or reproductive tract. In the initial evaluation of a horse with hematuria, signalment and clinical signs can significantly aid in the diagnosis. The diagnostic process should involve serum biochemical analysis, rectal

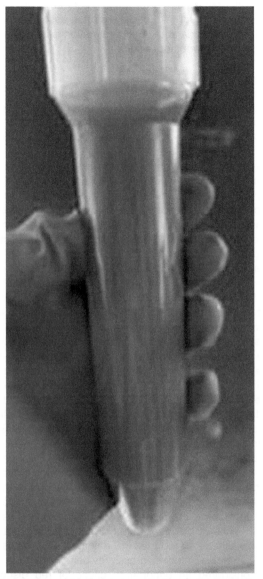

Fig. 1. Urine collected after exercise in a stakes-winning thoroughbred racehorse presented with recurrent hematuria after racing or breezing. The horse did not have hematuria at any other time, and his renal values, muscle enzymes (preexercise and postexercise), complete blood count, and imaging of the urinary tract were all within normal limits. The horse was healthy otherwise but continued to have intermittent hematuria after strenuous exercise.

palpation of the urinary and reproductive tract, imaging of the urinary structures (ultra-sonography and endoscopy), urinalysis, and sometimes bacterial culture.

Timing of the discoloration during micturition may be suggestive of the location of the lesion. Persistently discolored streams, from beginning to end of urination, are usually associated with hematuria owing to renal, ureteral, or bladder lesions. Discolored streams at the beginning of micturition are often associated with lesions in the distal urethra. Instead, hematuria at the end of urination is usually associated with lesions in the proximal urethra or bladder neck.

Causes of Hematuria

Exercise-induced hematuria. Hematuria, as well as pigmenturia (hemoglobinuria or myoglobinuria) and proteinuria, can be observed in horses after strenuous exercise.[3] The most common to rule out in cases of hematuria during or after exercise are cystoliths, which can be easily diagnosed by rectal palpation, ultrasonography, or cystoscopy.

Exercise-associated hematuria, unrelated to bladder calculi, is a well-described finding in human athletes. The prevalence seems to depend on the type of exercise.[4] Affected people are usually asymptomatic and otherwise healthy; the hematuria is generally microscopic and pronounced in the first urine voiding after exercise. It normalizes within 72 hours in most cases. The degree of hematuria seems to be related to the intensity of the exercise. Several pathophysiologic mechanisms have been hypothesized, among them direct urinary tract trauma (of the bladder against the pelvic brim, or in in-contact sports), and increased glomerular permeability occurring during exercise. The latter might have been the origin of microscopic hematuria in a large number of cases.[5] Little is known about treatment or prevention, but in human athletes exercising without a completely voided bladder and preventing dehydration by high fluid intake, even in the form of beer, may aid in prevention.[6,7]

Similarly, in horses, exercise-induced hematuria has been reported by Schott and colleagues.[3] In the study, the source of the hematuria seemed to be related to the upper urinary tract as the investigators sampled the urine bypassing the bladder by directly catheterizing the ureters. This seems to be in line with the human medicine findings, where the potential mechanism for the hematuria appears to be an alteration in one or more of the factors affecting filtration across the glomerular barrier.

Bladder trauma should also be considered as an inciting cause: Schott[8] reported a mare with macroscopic hematuria after exercise owing to bladder mucosa erosions secondary to direct trauma of the bladder against the pelvic rim during exercise. This cause has been reported in people and should be suspected especially when the bladder is voided right before exercise. A recent case report described a case of hemorrhagic cystitis in a horse where exercise intensity might have been the etiologic factor for the development of bladder-wall hyperplasia and hematuria.[9]

Another potential cause of bladder trauma to consider is protruding osteochondroma of the os pubis as recently reported in 2 geldings with exercise-induced hematuria.[10] Regardless, exercise-induced, grossly evident, hematuria not caused by a cystolith can be considered an uncommon cause of red discolored urine (see **Fig. 1**). Of note, because in most of the self-limiting equine and human cases reported, the hematuria is microscopic, macroscopic hematuria might indicate urinary dysfunction or trauma. Therefore, diagnostic investigation to rule out urinary or extraurinary disease is recommended. Hemoglobinuria or myoglobinuria might also occur following exercise and would need to be differentiated from hematuria.[3]

Urolithiasis

Postexercise hematuria is the most common clinical sign observed in horses with cystic calculi. Typically, the hematuria is evident near the end of urination. Male horses are more predisposed than female horses to cystic calculi. Pollakiuria, stranguria, incontinence, and urine dribbling might be observed for calculi present in the bladder or the urethra. Prolonged periods of penile protrusion and urine or blood staining on the hind limbs can also be present.

Cystic calculi can be confirmed by rectal palpation (likely to be detected with only the hand and wrist in the rectal cavity) and ultrasonography. In any case of uroliths, detailed imaging of the different urinary tract structures is recommended because of the frequent presence of calculi in multiple locations (almost 10% of horses with urolithiasis have multiple calculi in various locations of the urinary tract).[11] This suggests that nephroliths may play a leading role in the pathogenesis of urolithiasis. It is known that most ureteroliths are likely to start in the renal pelvis, and occasionally small uroliths can even reach the bladder. Nephroliths (**Fig. 2**) and ureteroliths are detected less commonly than cystic and urethral calculi. When present, they can produce a partial or complete obstruction. When found bilaterally and causing obstruction, signs of chronic renal failure might be present (azotemia, weight loss, isosthenuria). Mild recurrent colic might be the only clinical sign for unilateral nephroliths or ureteroliths. Evidence of microscopic hematuria on dipstick is commonly detected in these cases, and intermittent or persistent gross hematuria might also be seen.

Therapeutic procedures are based on the location and the size of the calculi. Because alkalotic pH is among the factors favoring the growth of the uroliths, the use of urine acidifiers (ammonium chloride, ammonium sulfate, ascorbic acid) is often recommended as further prevention. However, there are no studies comparing the likelihood of recurrence of calculi between horses that have or have not received urinary acidifiers, and it is not easy to acidify the urine of horses. In a recent study, ammonium sulfate at 175 mg/kg produced a urine pH 5.0 (below pH 6.5 calcium carbonate uroliths do not form) and together with a low calcium diet was reported to be effective in preventing new calculi formation in a single case of a horse with recurrent cystic calculi.[12] Extrapolating from other species, diets rich in omega-3 fatty acids might have a beneficial effect on preventing calcium-based calculi formation.[13]

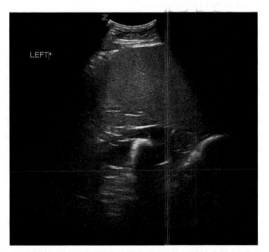

Fig. 2. A left nephrolith in the renal pelvis of a 15-year-old gelding presented for straining and discomfort owing to an obstructive urethral calculus that was removed surgically. Imaging of the left kidney revealed the presence of the nephrolith but no other abnormalities. The horse recovered well from surgery; no action was undertaken for the nephrolith, and the horse was reported to be well 2 years after presentation.

Urinary tract infection and pyelonephritis

Hematuria is a common clinical sign of UTI and is usually accompanied by dysuria, stranguria, pollakiuria, incontinence, urine scolding, and possibly also systemic signs of fevers and weight loss. When UTI is suspected, urinalysis and culture should be performed. The urine should be obtained by catheterization or midstream capture to avoid sampling of contaminants from the reproductive tract. Growth of more than 10,000 colony-forming units per milliliter of urine is often diagnostic of UTI. *Proteus mirabilis*, *Escherichia coli*, *Klebsiella* spp, and *Enterobacter* spp are among the most isolated pathogens in UTI cases. Gram-positive organisms are less frequently isolated. UTI can affect the lower urinary tract (bladder, urethra) or the upper urinary tract (kidneys, ureters). Multiparous mares are at a greater risk for lower UTI because of ascending infections secondary to injury at foaling. Horses with chronic atonic bladders are also predisposed. Pyelonephritis, infection involving renal pelvis and parenchyma, is a rare occurrence in horses and is often associated with the presence of nephroliths or ureteroliths. Fever, azotemia, polydipsia, polyuria, and abnormal leucogram findings are common clinical signs. Hematuria, macroscopic or microscopic, has been reported in cases of pyelonephritis. A case series of 7 horses with suspected pyelonephritis described the presence of unilateral or bilateral renal hemorrhage.[14] Overall, hematuria seems to be a common but not a consistent finding, and some pyelonephritis cases might have a recurrence of hematuria with time.[15] Treatment involves antibiotics based on urine culture and sensitivity, removal of predisposing factors (eg, calculi), and supportive care.

Idiopathic renal hematuria

Idiopathic renal hematuria (IRH) is characterized by acute onset of hemorrhage more commonly from 1 kidney but possibly from both. The hemorrhage can be life-threatening and, when profuse, blood clots might be passed. The pathophysiology remains unknown, hence the name idiopathic. Arabians seem to be predisposed, as more than 50% of the cases reported are Arabians or Arabian crosses. However, several other breeds have been affected, donkeys and mules included. No age or sex predisposition has been recognized.[16]

The diagnosis is reached excluding other causes of renal hemorrhage and hematuria. Upon cystoscopy, hemorrhage from one or both ureters is usually obvious. There is generally no evidence of UTI. The syndrome can present with initial mild episodes that might self-resolve but can reoccur with a hemorrhagic crisis. Because of similar features that this syndrome shares with pyelonephritis (abnormal ultrasound images, clinical signs), it has been hypothesized that they may represent the same pathologic condition.[17] In IRH cases as well as in some pyelonephritis cases, pyuria is absent, and cultures are negative. Treatment is largely supportive, involving blood transfusion when needed. Aminocaproic acid administration could also be beneficial in stopping the hemorrhage, reducing the fibrinolytic activity.

If the condition is unilateral, a nephrectomy might be resolutive; however, onset of bleeding from the contralateral kidney after nephrectomy has been reported.[15]

Neoplasia

Urinary neoplasia is a rare cause of hematuria. Nephroblastomas and adenocarcinomas are the most reported renal neoplasia, with the former being more common in younger animals and the latter being more common in older ones. Squamous cell carcinoma is the most common bladder tumor, followed by transitional cell carcinoma. Bladder neoplasias are more common in the older population. Lymphosarcoma, hemangiosarcoma, and melanoma rarely metastasize to the bladder, but may involve the renal tissue.

Clinical signs include hematuria, weight loss, discomfort, and occasionally pollakiuria and stranguria. This clinical presentation may closely resemble the one of cystic calculi with hematuria, stranguria, and a palpable mass on rectal examination. Ultrasonography and cystoscopy can be used to distinguish between the 2 conditions.

In cases of renal tumors, rectal palpation can reveal an enlarged kidney, especially if the left kidney is affected. Rectal and transabdominal ultrasound can reveal abnormal tissue or masses related to the kidneys. Urinalysis often shows hematuria. Urine cytology rarely reveals exfoliated neoplastic cells.

Treatment for a unilateral renal neoplasia is nephrectomy; unfortunately, often the tumor has already metastasized by the time the diagnosis is reached. A metastasis search should be carried out before surgical excision, as this would impact prognosis. For bladder neoplasms, surgical removal and topical chemotherapy might be attempted.[18]

Verminous nephritis

Halicephalobus gingivalis can be a rare cause of hematuria in horses owing to the formation of renal granulomas. The nematode can enter via mucous membranes, invade, and proliferate in several tissues, among which are the kidneys, central nervous system, long bones, and eyes. Affected horses can present with encephalitis, renal dysfunction, weight loss, hematuria, and/or polyuria. Classic lesions on the kidneys appear as multifocal large nodules. The granulomas might be visible on ultrasound, although the echogenicity might be similar to the cortical echogenicity and therefore difficult to localize. The nematode can occasionally be seen on urine sediment evaluation.[19] Treatment with a larvicidal anthelmintic can be attempted. Immediately after the treatment, signs of renal failure could occur because of inflammation caused by the death of the parasite; hence, simultaneous treatment with an anti-inflammatory is recommended.[15] Successful medical treatment has not been reported. If the lesion is only found in 1 kidney, a unilateral nephrectomy could be considered. Renal infection from *Strongylus vulgaris* has been reported in a foal,[20] as larval migration can involve the renal artery aberrantly.[21] *Dioctophyma renale* is a large nematode that could affect horses, although the typical hosts are carnivorous species, and cases in horses have not been reported. Adults can migrate and reach the kidneys and lay eggs that can be shed in the urine. Hydronephrosis and hematuria are occasional but serious complications of this infection.[22]

Idiopathic hemorrhagic cystitis

Primary hemorrhagic cystitis is a recently described cause of hematuria and stranguria in horses.[23] This syndrome is characterized by the presence of proliferative and hemorrhagic bladder mucosa detectable on cystoscopy. Hemorrhagic and thickened bladder mucosa affects more severely the apex of the bladder but can involve the entire bladder. The lesions might even resemble a proliferative mass depending on the individual case. Histopathology usually yields neutrophilic and hemorrhagic cystitis, but in some cases, could also reveal dysplasia or hyperplasia. These horses are generally otherwise healthy without specific hematological or biochemical findings apart from a possible mild anemia. The cause remains unknown; however, environmental, behavioral, viral, and drug-related causes have been hypothesized. Intense exercise was suggested as a potential cause in a recently reported case.[9] No evidence of bacterial growth in urine or bladder tissue has been reported. All the horses in the above-mentioned case series[23] were treated with trimethoprim-sulfa drugs and nonsteroidal anti-inflammatory drugs (NSAIDs) and recovered. It is difficult to conclude if they recovered because of the treatment. This syndrome can share several features with bladder neoplasia, such as history, clinical signs of hematuria and stranguria or pollakiuria, and evidence of abnormal bladder walls on ultrasound examination. Unlike horses with bladder neoplasia, horses with idiopathic hemorrhagic cystitis have a favorable prognosis. Histopathology and response to treatment can help differentiating the 2 conditions.

Nonsteroidal anti-inflammatory drugs–induced ulcerative cystitis

Hematuria owing to ulcerative cystitis has been reported in 2 horses treated with long-term phenylbutazone. In these horses, ulceration and hemorrhage of the urinary bladder were observed upon cystoscopy, and resolution of the hematuria was achieved after discontinuation of the NSAIDs and treatment with a prostaglandin analogue. No other causes for the cystitis were identified. The known adverse effects of NSAIDs treatment and the positive response after discontinuing the drug (confirmed on cystoscopy) suggested an association between phenylbutazone administration and ulcerative cystitis for these horses.[24] NSAIDs-induced cystitis should typically cause multifocal or diffuse lesions similar to cases of idiopathic hemorrhagic cystitis.

Long-term administration of NSAIDs can also induce necrosis of the renal medullary crest causing decreased medullary blood flow. Hyperechoic renal papilla and echogenic debris in the renal pelvis are characteristic ultrasonographic findings of renal medullary necrosis.[25]

Polypoid cystitis

Polypoid cystitis was recently reported as a cause of hematuria in a pony mare. On cystoscopy, multiple small pedunculated soft tissue structures were observed on the bladder mucosa. Histopathological analysis of the masses was consistent with chronic polypoid cystitis. Clinical signs and lesions resolved following prolonged antibiotic treatment.[26]

Urethral rents

Hematuria resulting from a urethral rent is usually detected at the end of urination because of the urethral contractions that occur at that stage.

The rent is usually located on the convex surface of the urethra at the level of the ischial arch and is usually linear and in correspondence with the corpus spongiosum (**Fig. 3**).[27] Stallions generally present with hemospermia and no gross hematuria, whereas geldings present with hematuria. The specific cause of urethral defects is not proved, but they might occur as a consequence of the dramatic increase in pressure in the corpus spongiosum at the end of urination in geldings or during ejaculation in stallions.

Urethral rents are diagnosed via endoscopy, and usually no inflammation surrounds the rent. These horses are usually otherwise healthy with no other specific clinical signs, but occasionally can present with dysuria. Blood work findings are normal or limited to mild anemia. Urinalysis might be normal if the urine is caught in early to midstream. Affected cases uncommonly might present perineal asymmetry or a widened perineum.[8]

Some rents heal without specific treatments; however, if the hematuria causes significant anemia or does not resolve, surgical treatment is indicated. Chemical cauterization with topical 4% policresulen solution has recently been reported as efficacious in some of these cases.[28]

Urethritis

Primary urethritis is not well documented in horses; however, occasionally hematuria and dysuria have been attributed to this condition. The prominent vasculature and

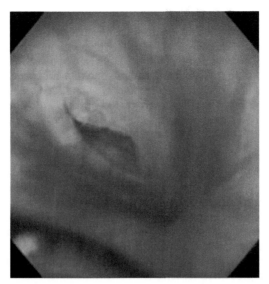

Fig. 3. A urethral rent on endoscopy in a quarter horse gelding presented for blood dripping at the very end of urination.

varicosities of the urethra can be easily mistaken on endoscopic examination for signs of local inflammation.[15] Nevertheless, traumatic, bacterial, neoplastic, or parasitic (*Habronema* infections) conditions can potentially cause primary urethritis.

Hematuria in foals

Gross hematuria is uncommon in foals. Differentials include trauma, urinary tract obstruction or rupture, toxicoses, drug-induced hematuria, sepsis, acute tubular necrosis, congenital malformations, and leptospirosis.

Complete physical examination, blood work, urinalysis and ultrasound evaluation of the abdominal cavity, and urinary structures are recommended to identify the source of hematuria. Because some umbilical abnormalities have been reported to be indirect causes of hematuria, imaging of the umbilical structures is recommended in the assessment of foals.

Cystic hematomas are reported as the cause of hematuria in a case series of 3 foals.[29] It has been hypothesized that trauma to the umbilicus during the periparturient period can result in damage to the umbilical vessels and the urachal sheath with retrograde bleeding into the proximal portion of the urachus, bladder, and umbilical arteries. This hemorrhagic process may then form a clot in the ventral portion of the bladder. These foals might present with gross hematuria only, but stranguria and discomfort can be present if the size of the hematoma is obstructive. Medical treatment with intravenous fluids in order to reduce the size of the clot and promote expulsion can be attempted. Surgical removal should be considered in cases of active hemorrhage or significative obstruction.

Nogradi and colleagues[30] reported an aortic aneurism and urethral obstruction secondary to umbilical artery abscessation as cause of hematuria in a 5-week-old foal. Similarly, a large abdominal abscess that had eroded into the right ureter was reported as cause of hematuria in a 4.5-month-old foal that eventually died owing to acute bleeding when the abscess eroded the aorta.[31] Congenital abnormalities as renal dysplasia and benign ureteropelvic polyps have been associated with hydronephrosis and hematuria.[32]

Specifically, congenital vascular abnormalities can also be a rare cause of hematuria. A recent report described a hamartoma of vascular origin causing chronic hematuria since birth in a 6-month-old Criollo. The hamartoma communicated with the lumen of the proximal urethra and led to progressive blood loss.[33] Congenital intrarenal arteriovenous fistula, congenital unilateral renal pseudoaneurysm, and pyelonephritis and extrarenal arterioureteral fistula (between an aortic aneurism and the left ureter) have been reported as causes of hematuria in foals.[34–36] Color-flow Doppler ultrasonography and advanced imaging with the use of angiography and contrast can aid in the diagnosis of vascular abnormalities.

Other causes of hematuria

Blister beetle toxicity causes gastrointestinal irritation and renal failure. Cantharidin, the toxin of blister beetles, is irritative to the urinary tract and may cause hemorrhage of the urinary mucosa. Microscopic or macroscopic hematuria can be noted during the progression of the toxicity. Cantharidin toxicity should be considered a differential diagnosis for horses that present with hematuria, gastrointestinal pain, oral erosions, and hypocalcemia and are fed alfalfa hay.

Chronic unilateral nephritis and vascular renal hypertension have been recently reported in a stallion presented for long-term intermittent hematuria. In this report, the cause of the initial nephritis was unclear; however, the acquired vascular anomalies seemed to have caused the hematuria.[37]

In young horses presenting with signs of acute renal disease, fevers, anorexia, and microscopic and/or macroscopic hematuria, leptospirosis should be considered, especially if more than 1 horse is affected on the same premises.

In horses presenting hematuria, intravascular hemolysis and acute renal failure, hemolytic uremic syndrome similar to the human syndrome caused by E coli verotoxins should be suspected.[15,38]

Any cause of uterine or vaginal bleeding could confound urinalysis and could be mistaken for hematuria. The source of hematuria can be confirmed via cystoscopy and urinalysis on urine samples obtained by catheterization.

Hematuria consequent to renal biopsy is common and can be present for several days at a macroscopic or microscopic level.

Hemoglobinuria

The presence of free hemoglobin in urine is defined as hemoglobinuria. The urine can appear clear to red-brown discolored depending on the hemoglobin concentration. Clinical presentation, with hematological and biochemical parameters, is key in differentiating hemoglobinuria from hematuria and myoglobinuria (**Fig. 4**). Intravascular hemolysis must be ongoing for the RBCs to lyse and release hemoglobin. As previously mentioned, the discoloration will not clear after centrifugation and sedimentation of the urine sample.

Patients with intravascular hemolysis will have pink/red discolored serum and can present with various clinical signs depending on the severity of the anemia, rate of RBCs destruction, and primary disease process. Pale mucous membrane, icterus, tachycardia, tachypnea, lethargy, and inappetence are among the most common clinical signs presented in moderate to severe cases regardless of the primary disease process. Various degrees of anemia, increased in serum protein concentration owing to the intravascular release of hemoglobin, increased bilirubin, and evidence of RBC regeneration (increased mean corpuscular volume [MCV]) are the common hematological findings.

Common causes of intravascular hemolysis and subsequent hemoglobinuria are parasitic (piroplasmosis), viral (equine infectious anemia), immune-mediated, or toxic.

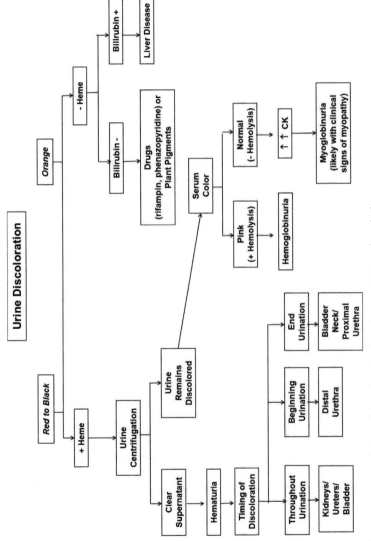

Fig. 4. Proposed diagnostic approach to red discolored urine. CK, creatinine phosphokinase.

Red maple leaf, phenothiazine, copper, and wild onion are the most common toxic causes, with hemolysis from red maple leaves toxicity being the most commonly reported in horses.[39]

Clostridium perfringens type A has been reported to have caused hemorrhagic gastritis, hemolysis, and renal failure in a horse. The hemolysis and hemoglobinuria were possibly due to the pathologic action of the alpha-toxin on erythrocytes cell membranes.[40]

The specific mechanism of hemoglobin-induced renal damage seems to be multifactorial involving direct damage to renal tubule cells, as free heme is a likely trigger of tubule barrier deregulation and oxidative cell damage. Furthermore, tubular obstruction with casts formed from cells debris, tubular cell necrosis directly caused by hemoglobin, and vascular constriction are described as direct damages from hemoglobin.[41]

Methemoglobinuria is another cause of discolored urine that produces brown-tinged color owing to high concentrations of methemoglobin. Methemoglobin is a hemoglobin in the form of metalloprotein formed by the reversible oxidation of heme iron to the ferric state instead of the ferrous state of normal hemoglobin. Methemoglobin cannot bind oxygen, and, when present in high quantities, also discolors the blood a bluish chocolate-brown. Nitrites and nitrates are reducing agents that can directly oxidize hemoglobin to methemoglobin. Red maple leaves, mint weed, and Sudan grass are some nitrate-accumulating plants that can cause methemoglobinemia if ingested either fresh or in forage.

Myoglobinuria

Myoglobinuria is the presence of myoglobin in urine. This is secondary to severe muscle injury (rhabdomyolysis) and damage to the cell membrane of the myocytes with consequent leakage of myoglobin into the plasma. The myoglobin is then filtered by the glomerulus and enters the renal tubular fluid. Horses that present with myoglobinuria have brown-to-red discolored urine and clinical signs of rhabdomyolysis, including stiffness, recumbency, colic, abnormal stance or gait, evidence of muscle pain, and swelling. Concentrations of creatinine phosphokinase and aspartate aminotransferase will be moderately to severely increased depending on the severity of the damage and its duration.

Common causes of muscular necrosis include traumatic myopathies, exertional myopathies, immune-mediated myopathies, postanesthetic myoneuropathies, atypical myopathy, clostridial myonecrosis, nutritional myodegeneration owing to selenium deficiency, and ingestion of toxins such as ionophores.[42]

The renal toxicity is due to contact of myoglobin with the tubules causing tubular necrosis and consequent renal failure. Three different mechanisms of renal toxicity by myoglobin are reported: renal vasoconstriction, formation of intratubular casts, and direct toxicity of myoglobin to renal tubular cells. Renal vasoconstriction can result from hypovolemia owing to excessive leakage of extracellular fluid into the damaged muscle cells and consequent activation of the renin-angiotensin-aldosterone system. The vasoconstriction could also be the result of myoglobin working as a nitric oxide scavenger and promoting cytokines release.[43] Intratubular casts formation is due to the interaction of myoglobin with the Tamm-Horsfall protein in the distal tubules. This process might be favored in the presence of acidic urine (rare in horses) and renal vasoconstriction.

Myoglobin contains iron as ferrous oxide, which is necessary for binding with oxygen. The oxidation of ferrous oxide to ferric oxide generates free hydroxyl radicals that can injure tubular epithelium and cause nephrotoxicity. Myoglobin itself can exhibit peroxidase-like enzyme activity and leads to lipid peroxidation. Therefore, a direct toxic effect of the myoglobin on the renal tubules, especially on the proximal tubules, is one of the mechanisms of direct renal injury.

In cases of myoglobinuria, the reagent strips will read positive for heme without been able to distinguish between myoglobin and other pigments. As previously mentioned, upon centrifugation, myoglobin does not sediment, and therefore, the urine will remain discolored. Clinical presentation and biochemical findings aid in the differentiation between hemoglobin and myoglobin; however, some specific tests can distinguish the 2 pigments. Ammonium sulfate precipitation can be helpful, as it indicates hemoglobin when precipitated at 80% saturation, whereas myoglobin gets precipitated only on full saturation. Direct spectrophotometry, centrifugation through a microconcentrator membrane, and electrophoresis are other methods able to distinguish the 2 pigments, but these are very rarely needed.

SUMMARY

This article reviewed common differentials for urine discoloration in horses and foals. The most common causes of hematuria are described, highlighting the different clinical presentations and diagnostic findings. The article also focused on the diagnostic process of differentiating hematuria from hemoglobinuria and myoglobinuria.

DISCLOSURE

The author has nothing to disclose.

REFERENCES

1. Ko DH, Jeong T-D, Kim S, et al. Influence of vitamin C on urine dipstick test results. Ann Clin Lab Sci 2015;45:391–5.
2. Coffman JR. Urinalysis. In: Coffman JR, editor. Equine clinical chemistry and pathophysiology. Bonner Springs (KS): Veterinary Medicine Publishing Company; 1981. p. 180–7.
3. Schott HC, Hodgson DR, Bayly WM. Haematuria, pigmenturia and proteinuria in exercising horses. Equine Vet J 1995;27:67–72.
4. Varma PP, Sengupta P, Nair RK. Post exertional hematuria. Ren Fail 2014;36: 701–3.
5. Akiboye RD, Sharma DM. Haematuria in sport: a review. Eur Urol Focus 2019; 5(5):912–6.
6. Ubels FL, van Essen GG, de Jong PE, et al. Exercise induced macroscopic haematuria: run for a diagnosis? Nephrol Dial Transplant 1999;14(8):2030–1.
7. Bassler TJ. Beer as prevention for runner's haematuria. Br Med J 1979;2(6200): 1293.
8. Schott HC. Discolored urine: causes you may have never considered. Intern Med Lame Pharmacol Physiol 2009;31:154–63.
9. Barton AK, Kershaw O, Gruber AD, et al. Equine idiopathic hemorrhagic cystitis: is it idiopathic or more likely to be exercise-associated? J Equine Vet Sci 2019; 78:6–9.
10. Rebsamen E, Geyer H, Furst A, et al. Hematuria in two geldings caused by osteochondroma of the os pubis: case reports and anatomic study of the os pubis in 41 cadaveric pelvises. Equine Vet Educ 2012;24:30–7.
11. Laverty S, Pascoe JR, Ling GV, et al. Urolithiasis in 68 horses. Vet Surg 1992;21: 56–62.

12. Remillard RL, Modransky PD, Welker FH, et al. Dietary management of cystic calculi in a horse. J Equine Vet Sci 1992;12:359–63.
13. Rodgers AL, Siener R. The efficacy of polyunsaturated fatty acids as protectors against calcium oxalate renal stone formation: a review. Nutrients 2020;12:1069.
14. Kisthardt KK, Schumacher J, Finn-Bodner ST, et al. Severe renal hemorrhage caused by pyelonephritis in 7 horses: clinical and ultrasonographic evaluation. Can Vet J 1999;40:571–6.
15. Schumacher J, Schumacher J, Schmitz D. Macroscopic haematuria of horses. Equine Vet Educ 2002;14:201–10.
16. Schott HC. Idiopathic renal hematuria. Diseases of the renal system. In: Smith B, editor. Large animal internal medicine. 5th editon. Maryland Heights (MD): Elsevier; 2015. p. 889–90.
17. Schumacher J, Schumacher J. Bloody urine - the list of differential diagnoses lengthens, but diagnostics remain the same. Equine Vet Educ 2019;31:255–9.
18. Divers TJ, Brault SA. Neoplasia disease of the renal system. In: Smith B, editor. Large animal internal medicine. 5th edition. Maryland Heights (MD): Elsevier; 2015. p. 885–6.
19. Kinde H, Mathews M, Ash L, et al. Halicephalobus gingivalis (H. deletrix) infection in two horses in southern California. J Vet Diagn Invest 2000;12:162–5.
20. Mahaffey LW, Adam NM. Strongylus vulgaris in the urinary tract of a foal and some observations upon the habits of the parasite. Vet Rec 1963;75:561–6.
21. Slocombe JO, Rendano VT, Owen RR, et al. Arteriography in ponies with Strongylus vulgaris arteritis. Can J Comp Med 1977;41:137–45.
22. Schott HC. Urinary tract infection and bladder displacement. In: Sprayberry KA, Robinson NE, editors. Robinson's current therapy in equine medicine. 7th edition. Philadelphia (PA): WB Saunders; 2014. p. 448–50.
23. Smith FL, Magdesian GK, Michel AO, et al. Equine idiopathic hemorrhagic cystitis: clinical features and comparison with bladder neoplasia. J Vet Intern Med 2013;32:1202–9.
24. Aleman M, Nieto JE, Higgins JK. Ulcerative cystitis associated with phenylbutazone administration in two horses. J Am Vet Med Assoc 2011;239:499–503.
25. Read WK. Renal medullary crest necrosis associated with phenylbutazone therapy in horses. Vet Pathol 1983;20:662–9.
26. Rosales CM, Bamford NJ, Sullivan SL, et al. Polypoid cystitis as a cause of haematuria in a pony mare. Equine Vet Educ 2019;31:250–4.
27. Schumacher J, Varner DD, Schmitz DG, et al. Urethral defects in geldings with hematuria and stallions with hemospermia. Vet Surg 1995;24:250–4.
28. Sancler-Silva YFR, Silva-Junior ER, Fedorka CE, et al. New treatment for urethral rent in stallions. J Equine Vet Sci 2018;64:89–95.
29. Arnold CE, Chaffin K, Rush BR. Hematuria associated with cystic hematomas in three neonatal foals. J Am Vet Med Assoc 2005;227:778–80.
30. Nogradi N, Magdesian KG, Whitcomb MB. Imaging diagnosis-aortic aneurysm and ureteral obstruction secondary to umbilical artery abscessation in a 5-week-old foal. Vet Radiol Ultrasound 2013;54:384–9.
31. Johnston JK, Neely DP, Latterman SA. Hematuria caused by abdominal abscessation in a foal. J Am Vet Med Assoc 1987;191:971–2.
32. Jones SL, Langer DL, Sterner-Kock A, et al. Renal dysplasia and benign ureteropelvic polyps associated with hydronephrosis in a foal. J Am Vet Med Assoc 1994;204:1230–1234s.

33. Busse NI, Paredes EA, Bustamante HA, et al. Periurethral vascular hamartoma in a 6-month-old foal with idiopathic hematuria: new differential diagnosis. J Vet Equine Sci 2018;67:19–22.
34. Schott HC II, Barbee DD, Hines MT, et al. Clinical vignette. Renal arteriovenous malformation in a quarter horse foal. J Vet Intern Med 1996;10:204–6.
35. Larsdotter S, Ley C, Pringle J. Renal pseudoaneurysm as a cause of hematuria in a colt. Can Vet J 2009;50:759–62.
36. Latimer FG, Magnus R, Duncan RB. Arterioureteral fistula in a colt. Equine Vet J 1991;23:483–4.
37. Garcia-Calvo LA, Duran ME, Martin-Cuervo M, et al. Persistent hematuria as a result of chronic renal hypertension secondary to nephritis in a stallion. J Equine Vet Sci 2014;34:709–14.
38. Dickinson CE, Gould DH, Davidson AH, et al. Hemolytic-uremic syndrome in a postpartum mare concurrent with encephalopathy in the neonatal foal. J Vet Diagn Invest 2008;20:239–42.
39. Alward A, Corriher CA, Barton MH, et al. Red maple (*Acer rubrum*) leaf toxicosis in horses: a retrospective study of 32 cases. J Vet Intern Med 2006;20:1197–201.
40. Patton K, Wright A, Kuroki K, et al. Hemorrhagic gastritis associated with renal failure, hemoglobinuria, and isolation of *Clostridium perfringens* in a horse. J Vet Equine Sci 2009;29:633–8.
41. Baines AD. Renal toxicity. Cambridge (MA): Blood substitutes Academic Press; 2006. p. 217–26.
42. Aleman M. A review of equine muscle disorders. Neuromuscul Disord 2008;18:277–87.
43. Blomberg LM, Blomberg MR, Siegbahn PE. A theoretical study of myoglobin working as a nitric oxide scavenger. J Biol Inorg Chem 2004;9:923–35.

Urinary Incontinence and Urinary Tract Infections

Tim Mair, BVSc, PhD, DEIM, DESTS, DipECEIM, AssocECVDI, FRCVS

KEYWORDS

- Urinary incontinence • Patent urachus • Ectopic ureter • Sabulous urolithisasis
- Bladder paralysis • Equine herpes virus myeloencephalopathy
- Cauda equina neuritis

KEY POINTS

- Urinary incontinence (the involuntary passage of urine) may result from primary disorders of the lower urinary tract (urinary bladder and urethra) or from neurologic diseases either of the nerve supply to the bladder/urethra or within the central nervous system.
- Congenital causes of urinary incontinence include patent urachus and ectopic ureter.
- Incontinence is typically diagnosed by the observation of constant or periodic dribbling of urine from the vulva or penis.
- Well-recognized neurologic causes of incontinence include equine herpes virus 1 myeloencephalopathy, polyneuritis equi (neuritis of the cauda equina), and sacral/coccygeal trauma.
- Idiopathic bladder paralysis is characterized by bladder paralysis and sabulous cystitis in the absence of overt neurologic deficits.

Urinary incontinence (the involuntary passage of urine) may result from primary disorders of the lower urinary tract (urinary bladder and urethra) or from neurologic diseases either of the nerve supply to the bladder/urethra or within the central nervous system (CNS). Functionally, micturition occurs in 3 phases:

- Bladder filling
- Postponement, comprising perception of the need to void urine, movement to a suitable place to urinate, adoption of voiding posture
- Voiding urine

Thus, micturition may be disturbed by intrinsic disease of the bladder or urethra, disorders of afferent or efferent nerve supply to the bladder/urethra, intracranial disease, or locomotor disturbance.

Although uncommon in horses, there are several different conditions that can present with incontinence.[1–3] However, distinguishing between them, as well as treating

---

Bell Equine Veterinary Clinic, CVS Ltd, Mereworth, Maidstone, Kent, ME18 5GS, UK
E-mail address: tim.mair@btinternet.com

Vet Clin Equine 38 (2022) 73–94
https://doi.org/10.1016/j.cveq.2021.11.006
0749-0739/22/© 2022 Elsevier Inc. All rights reserved.

vetequine.theclinics.com

them, can be very challenging.[4] Potential causes include congenital abnormalities, infectious diseases, traumatic injuries, and toxic insults (**Box 1**).[3] Urinary calculi have also been associated with incontinence in horses, especially mares, but will not be covered in this article (see "Surgery of the Equine Urinary Tract" in this issue).

CONGENITAL DISEASES
Patent Urachus

The urachus is the tubular structure that joins the fetal bladder to the allantois, and that allows fetal urine to drain into the allantoic cavity; it normally closes at birth, but failure to close at the time of parturition allows urine to leak from the urachus. The urachus remains persistently moist, and urine leaks as a drip or as a stream during micturition (**Fig. 1**). In some cases, urine leakage is not observed immediately after birth but becomes apparent within a few hours or days.[5–7] An excessively long or partially twisted umbilical cord has been proposed as a potential cause of patent urachus due to increased tension on the attachment of the umbilical cord to the body wall with subsequent dilation and failure to close at birth.[8] Septic omphalitis/omphalophlebitis can also predispose to a patent urachus within a few hours or days after birth; ultrasonographic examination can be helpful to distinguish between congenital patent urachus and acquired patent urachus associated with septic omphalitis.

Box 1
Causes of urinary incontinence in horses

Congenital causes
    Patent urachus and septic omphalitis/omphalophlebitis
    Ectopic ureter

Neurologic causes
    Sacral or coccygeal trauma
    Equine herpesvirus-1 myeloencephalopathy
    Equine protozoal myeloencephalopathy
    Equine degenerative myelopathy
    Equine motor neuron disease
    Cauda equina neuritis (polyneuritis equi)
    Neoplasia of the lumbosacral spinal cord
    Vertebral osteomyletitis and epidural empyema
    Parasitic myelitis

Idiopathic bladder paralysis
Trauma
    Foaling injuries and damage to the urethral sphincter

Cystolithiasis

Cystitis and urethritis

Hormonal
    Estrogen-responsive incontinence

Polyuria

Toxicities
    Sudan grass toxicity
    Sorghum cystitis ataxia

Iatrogenic
    Epidural administration of alcohol
    Iatrogenic damage to the urethral sphincter

Neoplasia

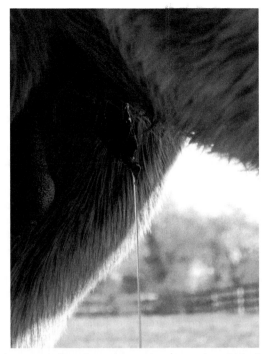

Fig. 1. Patent urachus. Urine flow from the urachus in a 3-day old foal.

A congenital patent urachus will normally close spontaneously within a few days in the absence of infection. Thus, no specific treatment is required. However, it is prudent to apply disinfectant solutions to the urachus to prevent secondary bacterial infection. Dilute chlorhexidine solution (0.5%) is more effective than 1% or 2% iodine solutions and is less irritant to the tissues.[9] The use of chemical cauterization, such as the application of phenol, 7% iodine, or silver nitrate is unnecessary and risks causing tissue necrosis, which may then predispose to bacterial infection.[9] Monitoring of the umbilicus using ultrasonography every 24 to 48 hours can be helpful in ensuring that the umbilicus is healing appropriately.[10] Although some clinicians advocate the routine use of antibiotics in foals with congenital patent urachus, this is likely unnecessary so long as the umbilicus is kept clean and monitored appropriately. If antibiotics are to be used, drugs that are eliminated in the urine (such as potentiated sulfonamides, aminoglycosides, or penicillins) are appropriate choices. Cephalosporins should be avoided unless indicated by culture and sensitivity results (due to their importance in human medicine).

In cases of acquired patent urachus associated with septic omphalitis/omphalophlebitis, broad-spectrum antibiotic therapy is indicated. Wherever possible, the choice of antibiotics should be based on the results of culture and sensitivity testing. Chemical cauterization is contraindicated because it increases the risk of urachal rupture and uroperitoneum.[11] In cases in which there is no improvement in urine leakage or where the ultrasonographic appearance shows no improvement after 5 to 7 days of medical treatment, then surgical resection of the urachus and umbilical vessels may be indicated.[12] A retrospective report of 33 foals with umbilical remnant infection found no differences in survival between foals treated with antibiotics and those treated with both antibiotics and surgery.[12] The decision to proceed to surgery should be made on a case-by-case basis, taking into account the risk of urachal rupture and development of uroperitoneum, or urachal leakage leading to cellulitis of the ventral abdominal wall and prepuce.[13]

ECTOPIC URETER

Ectopic ureter is rare but remains the commonest developmental abnormality of the equine urinary tract.[14] Although no breed predisposition has been identified, some investigators consider the Quarter Horse to be at greater risk.[15] The causes of ectopic ureter include failure of the ureteric bud to be incorporated into the urogenital sinus or failure to migrate cranial to the bladder neck, or failure of the mesonephric duct to regress. In the former, the ectopic ureter opens near the urethral papilla in females or into the pelvic urethra in males. In the latter, which only occurs in females, the ureter may open anywhere along the vagina, cervix, or uterus.[15] Most case reports (89%) of ectopic ureter in horses have been in females; however, this apparent sex predilection may reflect easier recognition of urinary incontinence in females (urine entering the urethra in males may pass retrograde into the bladder and therefore not result in consistent inappropriate voiding of urine).[15]

Urinary incontinence is often apparent from birth, and affected foals present with moisture and scalding on the hind limbs (**Fig. 2**). However, in some cases the condition may not be recognized for several months or years.[16] In cases of unilateral ectopia, affected foals will also void normal streams of urine because the other ureter opens normally into the bladder. Ultrasonography may show dilation of the affected ureter. Diagnosis can be achieved by endoscopic examination of the vagina and vestibule in females (while inflating the vagina with air and manually occluding the vulva) or the urethra in males. For the procedure, an endoscope is passed into the bladder and the ureteral ostia are identified. If one or both are absent, the endoscope is slowly withdrawn through the urethra so that the operator can look for the missing ostia. Intermittent urine flow is observed originating from the ectopic ureteral opening (usually from the area of the urethral papilla in females). Intravenous (IV) administration of dyes, such as sodium fluorescein (10 mg/kg IV), indigotindisulfonate (0.25 mg/kg IV), azosulfamide (2.0 mg/kg IV), or phenolsulfonphthalein (1.0 mg/kg IV), can help to identify the ectopic ureteral openings by discoloring the urine.[15] IV contrast urography, computed tomography, and scintigraphy can also be used for diagnosis.[17–19]

The only treatment options are surgical, including ureteral transposition and ureterocystostomy (surgical reimplantation of the ectopic ureter into the bladder) or unilateral nephrectomy. Before any surgical treatment, it must be established whether one or both ureters are ectopic and whether there are any other concurrent developmental abnormalities of the urogenital system.[20] Any preexisting urinary tract infection should be treated before surgical intervention. In the case of bilateral ectopic ureters (which were recorded in 8 of 20 cases by one investigator), the bladder volume and competency of the urethral sphincter should be assessed before surgery.[15] This assessment can be achieved by measuring the intravesicular pressure response to progressive distension until the infused fluid is voided. In 14 cases treated by ureterocystostomy , a successful outcome was reported in 10 cases, with 4 dying of postoperative complications.[15] In contrast, all 4 horses with unilateral ectopic ureters and treated by unilateral nephrectomy survived, so this treatment has been considered be more appropriate for such cases.[15] However, both ureteral transposition and ureterocystostomy , as well as unilateral nephrectomy, need to be performed under general anesthesia, and carry significant risks of morbidity. Recently, a minimally invasive technique of ureteral ostioplasty has been described in 2 fillies with unilateral ectopic

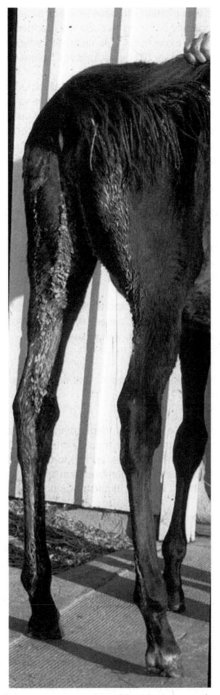

Fig. 2. Urine scalding of the perineum and hind legs in a 3-month-old filly with an ectopic ureter. (*Courtesy of* Dr T J Divers.)

ureter.[21] This procedure was possible in these 2 horses because the distended ureters could be seen cystoscopically coursing through the bladder wall, indicating that they were intramural rather than extramural. It is uncertain whether all ectopic ureters in horses are intramural, and this should be established before determining whether ureteral ostioplasty is feasible.

In dogs with ectopic ureter, urodynamic procedures including cystometrography to evaluate bladder capacity and detrusor function and urethral pressure profilometry to assess the urethral sphincter are routinely recommended before surgery because the most common postoperative complication is persistent incontinence.[16] Cystometrography has been reported before surgery in a few foals to document detrusor function and is appropriate to consider in future cases.[22,23]

EVALUATION OF URINARY INCONTINENCE IN ADULT HORSES

The diagnostic workup of a horse with urinary incontinence should include some or all the following:

- Clinical history (including any history of injury or musculoskeletal trauma, lameness, reproductive history in mares, etc)
- Musculoskeletal/lameness evaluation
- Neurologic evaluation
- Rectal palpation: assess the size and filling of the bladder, tone, and pain
- Transabdominal ultrasonography: assess the contents of the bladder (fluid/sediment), bladder wall, calculi, pelvic soft tissues
- Urethral catheterization
- Urethral and bladder endoscopy
- Blood analysis: hematology, fibrinogen, and serum amyloid A (SAA) concentrations, urea, creatinine
- Urinalysis and bacterial culture

Further examinations may be indicated, depending on the results of the history and previous examinations, such as viral polymerase chain reaction and serology, cerebrospinal fluid analysis, vitamin E analysis, and so forth. Radiographic and ultrasonographic examinations of the pelvis and lumbosacral spine may be helpful in cases of known or suspected trauma. Likewise, nuclear scintigraphy could be considered in selected cases.

Urodynamic tests can be used to assess how well the bladder and urethral sphincters function; these include cystometrography, urethral pressure profilometry, and simultaneous cystometry and uroflowmetry.[24,25] Urinary pressure profiling has been reported in horses, but it has rarely been described in the evaluation of incontinent horses.

NEUROLOGIC CONTROL OF MICTURITION

The bladder has 2 main functions: to store and to expel urine. Normal urination (maintenance of continence) requires a complex interaction between detrusor muscle activity (contractions) and urethral sphincter closure pressure controlled by the nervous system. This coordination of the lower urinary tract function depends on the interaction of both the sympathetic and parasympathetic system as well as somatic branches of the CNS (**Fig. 3**).[26–28] In bladder storage, the urethral closure pressure needs to exceed the pressure from detrusor (bladder) muscle contractions (ie, outflow resistance is high and detrusor tone is low). Normal voiding is achieved when urethral pressure decreases and bladder pressure increases. Problems with this mechanism and

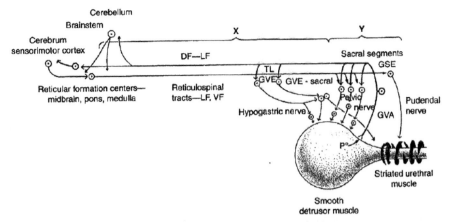

Fig. 3. Neuroanatomy of bladder function. Lesion at X: UMN lesion: Spinal cord reflex bladder. 1.No voluntary control: loss of bladder sensation. 2.Retention (brief)-distension-overflow. 3.Reflex micturition occurs with frequent voiding anywhere, initiated by abdominal pressure; slight residual remains. Lesion at Y: LMN lesion: Denervated bladder. 1.No voluntary control: loss of bladder sensation. 2.Retention-distension-overflow incontinence. 3.In time small, brief contractions of bladder muscle occur via an intramural reflex activity-incomplete-large residual remains. DF, dorsal funiculus; GSE, general somatic efferent; GVA, general visceral afferent; GVE, general visceral efferent; LF, lateral funiculus; TL, thoracolumbar; VF, ventral funiculus. (*From* De Lahunta A, Glass E, Kent M. Control of micturition. In: de Lahunta's Veterinary Neuroanatomy and Clinical Neurology. Philadelphia: Elsevier; 2021. p. 221-5; with permission.)

the coordination between urethral muscles and detrusor muscle can lead to incontinence.

Somatic innervation is primarily to the striated muscle of the urethra via a branch of the pudendal nerve, originating from the sacral spinal cord (S1-S4).[26–28] The sympathetic nerve supply comes from the hypogastric nerve, which originates from lumbar segments of the spinal cord (L1-L4), with the preganglionic fibers synapsing in the caudal mesenteric ganglion and postganglionic fibers supplying the bladder (primarily $\beta2$ receptors) and urethra (primarily $\alpha1$ and some $\alpha2$ adrenergic receptors). Parasympathetic innervation originates from the sacral cord (S2-S4) forming the pelvic nerve (these same segments also innervate the external genitalia and urethra).

During the storage (filling) phase, there is an increase in the tone of the smooth and striated muscles that form the external and internal urethral sphincters, which maintain continence; the pudendal nerve and sympathetic nerves innervate these muscles. During this phase, the smooth muscle of the bladder (the detrusor muscle) remains relaxed due to the influence of the pelvic nerve afferents and the sympathetic nerves innervating the muscle. The coordination of these actions is maintained by a reflex arc including bladder stretch and pressure receptors, afferent pelvic nerve, spinal cord interneurons, and sympathetic tone in hypogastric nerve efferents. The reflex allows the bladder to accumulate large volumes of urine with only small increases in intravesicular pressure. The tone of the urethral sphincters can also be mediated by upper motor neurons. Therefore, neurologic lesions anywhere in the spinal cord can result in bladder dysfunction.[3]

Intravesicular pressure increases once detrusor muscle fibers are fully stretched. Bladder wall receptors will detect this increase, stimulating sensory impulses to be sent via the pelvic nerve to the pons, cerebrum, and cerebellum, resulting in the sensation of bladder fullness. Voluntary micturition and emptying of the bladder are initiated by signals from the cerebrum and brainstem, which stimulate descending upper motor neurons (UMNs) in the reticulospinal tract to the sacral parasympathetic nuclei. Pelvic nerve impulses then stimulate detrusor muscle contraction, whereas stimulation of the pudendal and hypogastric sympathetic nerves results in relaxation of the urethral sphincters. The emptying phase ends when the bladder stretch receptors sense that the bladder is empty and afferent parasympathetic (pelvic nerve) impulses cease. Pelvic nerve efferent activity also ceases, and pudendal motor and sympathetic nerve activity resume, resulting in detrusor muscle relaxation.

Neurologic causes of urinary incontinence can result from 1 of 2 general forms: either dysfunction of UMN or lower motor neurons (LMN).[26–28] Disinhibition of the urethral sphincters resulting in increased urethral resistance can be caused by UMN disease, usually deep spinal cord lesions anterior to the pelvic ganglion. Damage to the LMN, on the other hand, results in paralysis of the detrusor muscle and an atonic bladder. LMN damage may arise in the sacral spinal cord segments, sacral spinal nerves, pelvic nerves and sacral plexus, or pudendal nerves.[27] The collection of nerves at the end of the spinal cord is known as the cauda equina, due to its resemblance to a horse's tail (Fig. 4). Damage to this region is a common cause of LMN damage resulting in urinary incontinence. Although distinguishing between UMN and LMN causes of incontinence may seem important, in reality the treatment and management of affected horses is often the same, regardless of the underlying cause.

CLINICAL SIGNS OF NEUROLOGIC BLADDER DYSFUNCTION

Incontinence is typically diagnosed by the observation of constant or periodic dribbling of urine from the vulva or penis.[28] In many cases, bladder dysfunction may have been present for a variable period of months to years before these signs are noticed by owners. Scalding of the skin and associated alopecia and accumulation of calcium carbonate deposits of the hind limbs (Fig. 5), perineum (in mares), and ventral abdomen (in males) often occurs in chronic cases. Urine may also be involuntarily voided in association with exercise and coughing or other activities that result in an increase in intra-abdominal pressure.

UMN bladder dysfunction results from lesions cranial to the sacral segments that interrupt the cranially projecting sensory and caudally projecting motor pathways.[27] UMN disease is characterized by increased urethral pressure, which may make urinary catheterization difficult, but horses affected by UMN disease often present with other severe neurologic signs, such as recumbency, which dominate the clinical

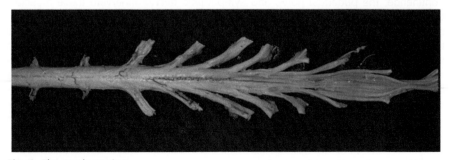

Fig. 4. The cauda equina.

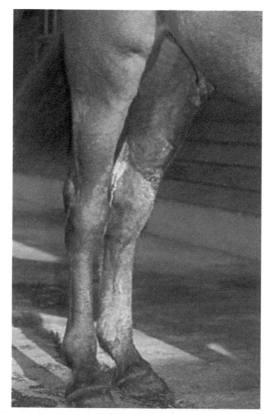

Fig. 5. Urine scalding of the skin of the hind limbs secondary to urinary incontinence.

management of the case. If these other clinical problems associated with UMN disease are manageable then the affected horse may develop the ability to urinate reflexively[7]; this is characterized by frequent urination, especially when there is an increase in intra-abdominal pressure, for example, during exercise. The bladder is often not completely emptied, which may result in deposits of sabulous material, similar (but not usually as severe) to horses affected by LMN bladder paralysis. Urine dribbling often occurs intermittently as well. Potential treatments for UMN bladder dysfunction could include sympatholytic drugs such as phenoxybenzamine, acepromazine, or prazosin to block the sympathetic alpha-1 receptors in the smooth muscle of the internal sphincter; parasympathomimetic drugs like bethanechol to stimulate the detrusor muscle; and skeletal muscle relaxants like benzodiazepines or dantrolene to block the striated urethralis muscle.[27]

LMN disease causes bladder paralysis and is often accompanied by other signs of sacral or lumbosacral dysfunction, such as loss of external anal sphincter tone (**Fig. 6**), reduced or absent perineal reflex, tail paralysis, analgesia or hypalgesia of the perineum, atrophy of the muscles of the hip and hind limb, and paresis of the hind limbs. Occasionally, the penis or vulva may also appear paralyzed (**Fig. 7**). The bladder distends with urine, and urine continually overflows and dribbles from the urethral orifice. The bladder can usually be evacuated by putting pressure on it per rectum; the only resistance to this will be at the internal urethral sphincter.

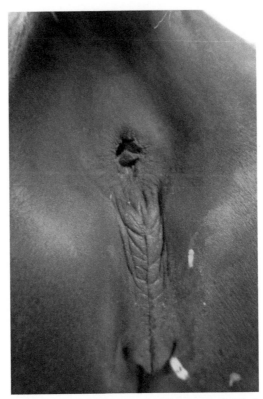

Fig. 6. Loss of external anal sphincter associated with sacrocaudal dysfunction.

NEUROLOGIC CAUSES OF URINARY INCONTINENCE

Well-recognized neurologic causes of incontinence include equine herpes virus 1 myeloencephalopathy,[3,29–32] polyneuritis equi (neuritis of the cauda equina),[33–35] and sacral/coccygeal trauma.[36] Lumbosacral intervertebral disk protrusion has also been reported as a cause of urinary incontinence.[37]

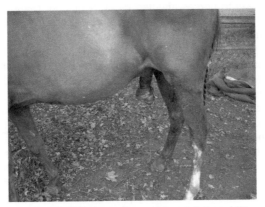

Fig. 7. Urine scalding of the hind limbs and paraphimosis in a gelding.

Equine herpesvirus-1 (EHV-1) infection is ubiquitous in most horse populations throughout the world and causes disease in horses and extensive economic losses through frequent outbreaks of respiratory disease, abortion, neonatal foal death, and myeloencephalopathy.[38] Myeloencephalopathy is an uncommon manifestation of EHV-1 infection; occasionally it has also been associated with EHV-4 infection. The clinical signs are the result of multifocal vasculitis, hemorrhage, thrombosis, and ischemia in the spinal cord.[39] Clinical signs, which commonly follow an episode of fever or coughing in the affected horse or in its in-contact herd mates, include sudden onset and stabilization of signs of ataxia, paresis, and urinary incontinence. Single or multiple cases may occur on the premises, and infection may be spread by horses attending external shows and events.[39–41] Most EHV-1 infections that cause neurologic disease represent reinfection rather than recrudescence of a chronic infection, and infection is usually in horses with significant preexisting serum antibody titers. Those horses that develop myeloencephalopathy are usually the ones that show the most rapid increases in antibody titers after infection. The onset of neurologic signs may or may not have been preceded by signs of upper respiratory tract disease, fever, or hind limb edema during the previous 2 weeks.[42] The diagnosis and management of equine herpes myeloencephalopathy are beyond the scope of this article, and readers are referred to other sources of information on these topics.[43]

The cause of polyneuritis equi is unknown, although both primary immunologic reaction and viral inflammatory disease have been suggested. The pathologic lesions resemble Guillain-Barre syndrome in man and experimental allergic neuritis in rodents (**Fig. 8**).[44] Initial clinical signs may include perineal hyperesthesia (presenting as tail and perineal pruritus) and hypalgesia/analgesia (**Fig. 9**), followed by progressive paralysis of the tail (**Fig. 10**), rectum, anus, and bladder (**Fig. 11**). Penile prolapse and urine dribbling may be seen in males.[33–35] Muscle atrophy of the gluteals and hind leg muscles (frequently asymmetric) may occur (**Fig. 12**). Asymmetric cranial nerve signs, including paralysis of the masticatory and facial muscles, head tilt, nystagmus, tongue paralysis, and dysphagia, may be observed.[26] There is no specific diagnostic test currently available. Cerebrospinal fluid analysis may show xanthochromia with mildly increased cell counts and total protein concentrations.[34] Definitive diagnosis is made by postmortem examination. There is currently no effective treatment, although corticosteroids may result in some temporary improvement.

The spectrum of neurologic diseases accompanied by incontinence may also include horses afflicted with equine protozoal myeloencephalitis, cervical stenotic

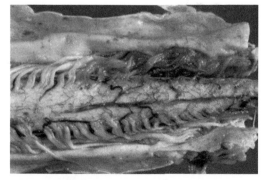

Fig. 8. Cauda equina neuritis (polyneurits equi). Postmortem appearance of the cauda equina showing chronic inflammatory changes.

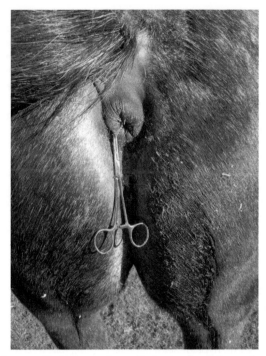

Fig. 9. Cauda equina neuritis (polyneurits equi). Analgesia of the perineum.

myelopathy, and equine degenerative myelopathy.[3] Although the latter 2 diseases do not directly affect the sacral segments, bladder paralysis, overflow incontinence, and sabulous urolithiasis have been recognized in some affected horses.

Neoplastic infiltration of the lumbosacral spine is an infrequent cause of urinary incontinence, usually associated with other clinical signs such as fecal incontinence, reduced tail tone, weakness, lameness, and muscle atrophy. Melanoma in gray horses is the commonest neoplasm that can present in this fashion, but other rarer tumors and other nonneoplastic infiltrative lesions (such as pyogranulomatous lesions) can also cause similar signs.[45–47]

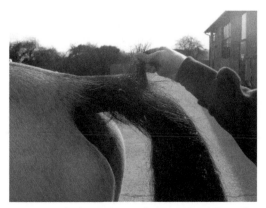

Fig. 10. Cauda equina neuritis (polyneurits equi). Paralysis of the tail.

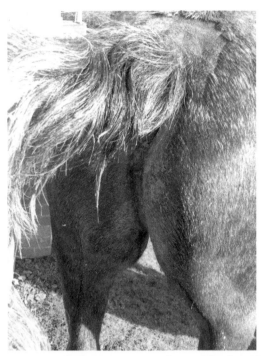

Fig. 11. Cauda equina neuritis (polyneurits equi). Urine and fecal scalding of the perineal skin due to urinary and fecal incontinence.

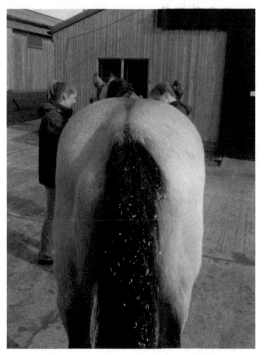

Fig. 12. Cauda equina neuritis (polyneurits equi). Asymmetric muscle atrophy.

IDIOPATHIC BLADDER PARALYSIS

Idiopathic bladder paralysis is characterized by bladder paralysis and sabulous cystitis in the absence of overt neurologic deficits.[3,48–50] It seems probable that a proportion of cases diagnosed with idiopathic bladder paralysis have an underlying neurologic initiating cause, but there are no other identifiable signs of neurologic dysfunction; in other words, prior neurologic disease cannot be ruled out with confidence.[3] Over time, the chronic distension of the bladder and the accumulation of heavy deposits of sabulous material likely cause myogenic detrusor damage, which perpetuates the bladder dysfunction (**Fig. 13**). Sabulous urolithiasis is the term used to describe accumulation of urine sediment, primarily calcium carbonate crystals, in the ventral aspect of the bladder (**Fig. 14**).[3,48–50] The accumulated urine sediment can develop into a large, inspissated mass (**Fig. 15**), which on initial palpation per rectum may be mistaken for a cystolith; however, the concurrent finding of a large, atonic bladder should alert the clinician to consider bladder paralysis and sabulous urolithiasis.[49,50] In contrast, cystoliths are usually found in small bladders, and incontinence is often accompanied by stranguria, which is absent in cases of bladder paralysis. Despite recognition for several centuries, the syndrome of bladder paralysis, complicated by urinary incontinence and sabulous urolithiasis, remains poorly understood.[12] A major reason for this lack of understanding is the fact that affected horses may not present for months to years after onset of the problem that eventually leads to incontinence. Therefore, the clinician is often faced with the end stage of the syndrome when horses are initially presented for evaluation of incontinence.[49,50]

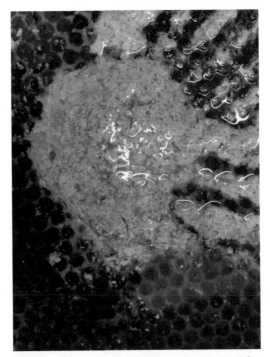

Fig. 13. Heavy deposit of calcium carbonate in the urine drained from the bladder of a horse with sabulous urolithiasis.

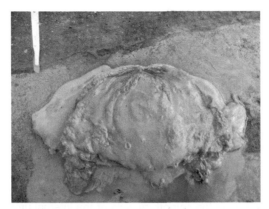

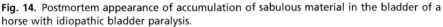

Fig. 14. Postmortem appearance of accumulation of sabulous material in the bladder of a horse with idiopathic bladder paralysis.

In some cases, urinary incontinence may arise secondary to mild neurologic disease or musculoskeletal problems that prevent the normal posturing for urination. The identification of mild neurologic causes of bladder dysfunction may be difficult in the absence of the more overt clinical signs associated with polyneuritis equi. However, 50% of cases of sabulous urolithiasis in one report had a variety of neurologic deficits, including perineal hypalgesia, various degrees of ataxia, and impaired proprioception.[49] In another review of urinary incontinence, 11 of 37 cases had either neurologic disease or detectable neurologic lesions at postmortem examination.[3]

Chronic accumulation of urine and sabulous deposits of calcium carbonate crystals in the bladder lead to detrusor muscle atony. The weight of the accumulated urine and sabulous deposits leads to stretching of the detrusor muscle and inability to contract. Eventually the ability to maintain sphincter function is lost and incontinence develops.

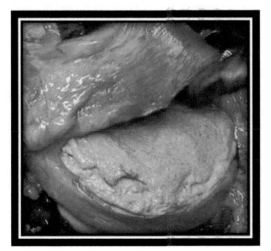

Fig. 15. Postmortem appearance of a mass of sabulous material in the bladder of a horse with idiopathic bladder paralysis. (*Courtesy of* Dr T J Divers.)

The accumulation of sediment and retention of urine with production of ammonia irritate the mucosa of the bladder and cause secondary cystitis, which further damage the bladder musculature.

Treatment of bladder paralysis should aim to assist urine evacuation to avoid detrusor atony from chronic overdistension of the bladder.[27] Bladder lavage is often successful at removing the accumulated sediment, although in some cases sediment may be firmly adherent to areas of bladder mucosal ulceration. Repeated lavage will be required to remove the sabulous material as it continues to be deposited over time. An indwelling urinary or Foley catheter can accomplish this but is often impractical in the long term due to ascending infection resulting in bacterial cystitis. Pharmacologic treatments may include bethanechol, a direct-acting parasympathomimetic drug, to stimulate the muscarinic receptors in the detrusor muscle.[27,51] In dogs, phenoxybenzamine or prazosin, alpha-adrenergic blockers, are used to block the sympathetic alpha-1 receptors in the smooth muscle of the internal urethral sphincter, but these have not been described in the horse. It is likely that any pharmacologic treatment would need to be instituted early in the disease process to be effective to avoid permanent detrusor dysfunction.

Bacterial cystitis and ascending urinary tract infection resulting in uretitis, pyelonephritis, and interstitial nephritis with renal failure can occur secondary to idiopathic bladder paralysis or cauda equina neuritis.[52,53] Clinical signs may include chronic weight loss, anorexia, apathy, and depression. Complementary laboratory and sonographic assessment can be helpful to confirm renal involvement. The prognosis is poor.

There have been few reports of the long-term outcomes of horses affected by idiopathic bladder paralysis; most horses require euthanasia due to problems associated with chronic/recurrent cystitis and/or ascending urinary tract infection. Rendle and colleagues[51] reported the outcomes of 5 horses with sabulous cystitis that were managed for up to 3 years. The horses were treated by emptying the bladder through a urinary catheter and saline lavage with cystoscopic guidance to remove residual sabulous material. The cystitis was treated with antimicrobial and anti-inflammatory medications, and bethanechol chloride was also administered. Frequent catheterization and emptying of the bladder were an alternative to regular cystoscopic examination with saline lavage, but this resulted in the development of a urethral stricture in one case. Four of the horses returned to work, and one was retired owing to persistent incontinence.

TRAUMA: DAMAGE TO THE URETHRAL SPHINCTER

Damage to the urethral sphincter can occur in mares secondary to foaling or breeding injuries. It is possible that pregnancy and parturition may be an underrecognized cause of urinary incontinence in multiparous mares. A history of dystocia, even several years previously, should be considered a potential inciting cause in mares presenting for evaluation of incontinence.[16,54] Iatrogenic damage can also occur as a result of surgical procedures, such as removal of cystic calculi or accidental damage caused by a vaginal speculum.[55,56] Surgical repair of the damaged sphincter by apposition of the ends of the ruptured or transected urethralis muscle and tunica muscularis may be possible in some cases.[55] Urethral rupture in males can rarely occur secondary to urethral calculus obstruction or direct trauma (eg, a kick); urinary incontinence can follow, associated with urine leakage into the periurethral soft tissues and tissue necrosis (**Fig. 16**). Paraphimosis in males can also present with urinary incontinence, depending on the underlying cause.

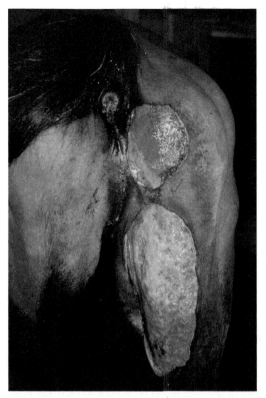

Fig. 16. Extensive skin necrosis secondary to urethral rupture in a gelding.

CYSTITIS AND URETHRITIS

Cystitis and chronic urethritis can result in urinary incontinence due to irritation of stretch receptors in the bladder wall resulting in stimulation of parasympathetic afferents and stimulation of detrusor contractions, which cannot be inhibited voluntarily[27]; this results in an apparent increase in the frequency of urination (pollakiuria) and an inability to control when the urination occurs. This condition is sometimes called "urge incontinence" due to detrusor overactivity. This situation may also arise in cases of unilateral ectopic ureter where the bladder is smaller than normal (due to disuse) and therefore incapable of storing normal volumes of urine.

Cystitis in horses is often secondary to other diseases of the lower urinary tract such as cystic calculi and UMN or LMN bladder dysfunction. Frequent catheterization to relieve bladder distension (for example, in cases of equine herpes myeloencephalopathy or atypical myopathy) can predispose to cystitis. Neoplasia is rare in the urinary bladder but can also result in secondary cystitis. Ulcerative cystitis has also been reported in horses receiving long-term phenylbutazone therapy.[57] Diagnosis and investigation of cystitis should include cystoscopy (**Fig. 17**) and urinalysis midstream voided or catheterized sample submitted for cytology and quantitative culture; generally the colony count of the offending organisms will be $\times 10^4$ colony-forming units/mL of urine or greater. Antibiotic therapy should be based on culture and sensitivity results, and the ability of the antibiotic to concentrate in the urine, as well as practical considerations, such as cost, ease of administration, and toxicity.

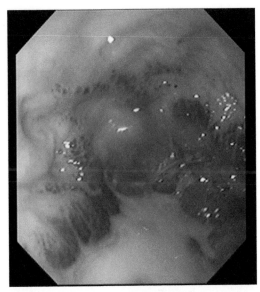

Fig. 17. Cystoscopy showing inflamed/hemorrhagic bladder mucosa in cystitis.

ESTROGEN-RESPONSIVE URINARY INCONTINENCE

Estrogen-responsive urinary incontinence ("hypoestrogenism") has been reported as a cause of urinary incontinence in a small number of mares.[3,58,59] Estrogen may increase the sensitivity of urethral alpha receptors to increase internal sphincter tone. In one case, an 18-year-old Shetland Pony mare responded to small doses (2 mg intramuscularly every 48 hours) of estradiol cypionate.[58] Another 2 mares were reported to have estrogen-responsive urinary incontinence.[59] The dose of estradiol benzoate administered to one of these mares (6 mg intramuscularly for 3 days and then alternate day treatments) was 3 to 6 times in excess of that expected to produce physiologic estrous levels. In contrast, the second mare responded to very low exogenous levels of estradiol, which corresponded to physiologic estrous concentrations (5 mg intramuscularly for 4 days, then every third day, and was subsequently maintained on 2.5 mg intramuscularly every third day).[59]

POLYURIA

Conditions resulting in severe polydipsia and polyuria (such as diabetes insipidus) have been reported to cause urinary incontinence as a result of chronic bladder dilatation, enuresis, and bladder overflow.[60]

TOXICITIES

Cystitis and caudal limb ataxia can occur in horses grazing pastures containing species of sorghum, especially hybrid crosses of sorghum (*Sorghum vulgare*) and Sudan grass (*S vulgare var sudanense*), and Johnson grass (*Sorghum halepense*).[61] The toxic principle is believed to be associated with the development of cyanide in the plant during periods of rapid growth; well-cured hay does not appear to be toxic. Cases have been reported in the western and southwestern states of the United States and Australia.[61–63] The clinical signs include symmetric ataxia, hind limb weakness, flaccid paralysis of the tail, and urinary incontinence. On rectal examination, hard concretions of sabulous material may be identified in the bladder. A bunny-hopping gait is sometimes seen. Treatment is supportive with removal from the source of the toxin.

DISCLOSURE

No commercial or financial conflicts of interest. No funding.

REFERENCES

1. Berger S. Urinary incontinence in the horse: 19 cases. [German] Harninkontinenz beim Pferd. Wiener Tierarztliche Monatsschrift 2011;98:66–75.
2. Schott, H. C., II. Unusual urinary tract disease syndromes: incontinence and urethrolithiasis. Proc. 31st Bain GFallon memorial lectures: internal medicine, lameness, pharmacology, physiology, Twin Waters Resort, Queensland (Australia). August 2009;31:164–74.
3. Schott HC II, Carr EA, Patterson JS, et al. Urinary incontinence in 37 horses. Proc 50th Ann Conv Am Assoc Equine Pract. Denver (CO). December 2004;50:345–47.
4. Guidi E, Nolf M, Cadore JL. Diagnosis and therapy of equine urinary incontinence. [French] L'incontinence urinaire chez le cheval: demarche diagnostique et therapeutique. Le Nouveau Praticien Veterinaire – Equine 2011;26:17–22.
5. Turner TA, Fessler JF, Ewert KM. Patent urachus in foals. Eq Pract 1982;4:24–5.
6. Richardson DW. Urogenital problems in the neonatal foal. Vet Clin North Am Equine Pract 1985;1:179–88.
7. Robertson JT, Embertson RM. Surgical management of congenital and perinatal abnormalities of the urogenital tract. Vet Clin North Am Equine Pract 1988;4:359–79.
8. Whitwell KE. Morphology and pathology of the equine umbilical cord. J Reprod Fertil Suppl 1975;23:599–603.
9. Lavan RP, Madigan J, Walker R, et al. Effects of disinfectant treatments on the bacterial flora of the umbilicus of neonatal foals. Biol Reprod Monog 1995;1:77–85.
10. Reef VB, Collatos C. Ultrasonography of umbilical structures in clinically normal foals. Am J Vet Res 1988;49:2143–6.
11. Ford J, Lokai MD. Ruptured urachus in a foal. Vet Med Small Anim Clin 1982;77:94–5.
12. Reef VB, Collatos C, Spencer PA, et al. Clinical, ultrasonographic, and surgical findings in foals with umbilical remnant infections. J Am Vet Med Assoc 1989;195:69–72.
13. Lees MJ, Easley KJ, Sutherland JV, et al. Subcutaneous rupture of the urachus, its diagnosis and surgical management in three foals Equine. Vet J 1989;21:462–4.
14. Baker JR, Ellis CE. A survey of post mortem findings in 480 horses 1958-1980: (1) causes of death Equine. Vet J 1981;13:43–6.
15. Schott HC, Waldridge B, Bayly WM. Disorders of the urinary system. Anatomy and development. In: Reed SM, Bayley WM, Sellon DC, editors. Equine internal medicine. 2nd edition. St. Louis (MO): Elsevier; 2018. p. 888–98.
16. Schott HC. Ectopic ureter - a leaky problem no matter how you look at it! Equine Vet Educ 2011;23:603–5.
17. Coleman MC, Chaffin MK, Arnold CE, et al. The use of computed tomography in the diagnosis of an ectopic ureter in a Quarter Horse filly. Equine Vet Educ 2011;23:597–602.

18. Leglise AS, Courouce-Malblanc A, Maurin E, et al. Diagnosis of an ectopic ureter in a nine-year-old filly using intravenous urography. (Special issue: Neurologie) [French] Diagnostic d'un uretere ectopique par urographie intraveineuse chez une ponette. Pratique Vet Equine 2004;36:53–9.
19. Getman LM, Ross MW, Elce YA. Bilateral ureterocystostomy to correct left ureteral atresia and right ureteral ectopia in an 8-month-old standardbred filly. Vet Surg 2005;34:657–61.
20. Hahn K, Conze TM, Wollanke B, et al. Urogenital hypoplasia and X chromosome monosomy in a draft horse filly. J Eq Vet Sci 2021;96:103318.
21. Jones ARE, Ragle CA. A minimally invasive surgical technique for ureteral ostioplasty in two fillies with ureteral ectopia. J Am Vet Med Assoc 2018;253:1467–72.
22. Christie B, Haywood N, Hilbert B, et al. Surgical correction of bilateral ureteral ectopia in a male Appaloosa foal. Aust Vet J 1981;57:336–40.
23. Squire KRE. Adams SB Bilateral ureterocystostomy in a 450-kg horse with ectopic ureters. J Am Vet Med As 1992;201:1213–5.
24. Ronen N. Measurements of urethral pressure profiles in the male horse. Equine Vet J 1994;26:55–8.
25. Kay AD, Lavoie JP. Urethral pressure profilometry in mares. J Am Vet Med Assoc 1987;191:212–6.
26. Furr M, Sampieri F. Differential diagnosis of urinary tract incontinence and cauda equine syndrome. In: Furr M, Reed S, editors. Equine Neurology. Ames (IA): Blackwell Publishing; 2008. p. 119–25.
27. De Lahunta A, Glass E, Kent M. Control of micturition. In: de Lahunta's veterinary neuroanatomy and clinical Neurology. Philadelphia (PA): Elsevier; 2021. p. 221–5.
28. Bayly WM. Urinary incontinence and bladder dysfunction. In: Reed SM, Bayley WM, Sellon DC, editors. Equine internal medicine. 2nd edition. St. Louis (MO): Elsevier; 2018. p. 973–90.
29. Friday PA, Scarratt WK, Elvinger F, et al. Ataxia and paresis with equine herpesvirus type 1 infection in a herd of riding school horses. J Vet Intern Med 2000;14:197–201.
30. Pusterla N, Hussey GS. Equine herpesvirus 1 myeloencephalopathy. Vet Clin North Am Equine Pract 2014;30:489–506.
31. Pusterla N, Hatch K, Crossley B, et al. Equine herpesvirus-1 genotype did not significantly affect clinical signs and disease outcome in 65 horses diagnosed with equine herpesvirus-1 myeloencephalopathy. Vet J 2020;255:105407.
32. Wilson WD. Equine herpesvirus myeloecephalopathy. Vet Clin North Am Equine Pract 1997;13:53–72.
33. Mair TS. Neuritis of the cauda equina in the horse. Vet Annu 1990;30:190–5.
34. Wright JA, Fordyce P, Edington N. Neuritis of the cauda equine in the horse. J Comp Pathol 1987;97:667–75.
35. Cummings J, Lahunta A, Timoney J. Neuritis of the cauda equine: a chronic idiopathic polyradiculoneuritis of the horse. Acta Neuropathol 1979;46:17–24.
36. Jeffcott LB. Disorders of the thoracolumbar spine of the horse – a survey of 443 cases. Equine Vet J 1980;12:197–210.
37. Krueger CR, Gold J, Barrett MF, et al. Diagnosis of lumbosacral intervertebral disc disease and protrusion in a horse using ultrasonographic evaluation and computed tomography. Equine Vet Educ 2016;28:685–9.
38. Lunn DP, Davis-Poynter N, Flaminio MJBF, et al. Equine herpesvirus-1 consensus statement. J Vet Intern Med 2009;23:450–61.
39. Reed SM, Toribio RE. Equine herpesvirus 1 and 4. Vet Clin North Am Equine Pract 2004;20:631–42.

40. Patel JR, Heldens J. Equine herpesviruses 1 (EHV-1) and 4 (EHV-4) – epidemiology, disease and immunoprophylaxis: a brief review. Vet J 2005;170:6–7.

41. Henninger RW, Reed SM, Saville WJ, et al. Outbreak of neurologic disease caused by equine herpesvirus-1 at a university equestrian center. J Vet Intern Med 2007;21:157–65.

42. McCartan CG, Russell MM, Wood JL, et al. Clinical, serological and virological characteristics of an outbreak of paresis and neonatal foal disease due to equine herpesvirus-1 on a stud farm. Vet Rec 1995;136:7–12.

43. Aleman M, Nout-Lomas YS, Reed SM. Disorders of the neurologic system. In: Reed SM, Bayley WM, Sellon DC, editors. Equine internal medicine. 2nd edition. St. Louis (MO): Elsevier; 2018. p. 580-708.

44. Kadlubowski M, Ingram PL. Circulating antibodies to the neuritogenic myelin protein, P2, in neuritis of the cauda equina of the horse. Nature 1981;293:299–300.

45. Hepworth-Warren KL, Wong DM, Galow-Kersh NL, et al. Metastatic tumor in pregnancy: placental germ cell tumor with metastasis to the foal. J Equine Vet Sci 2014;34:1134–9.

46. Portier K, Launois T, Desbrosse F. Cauda equina syndrome due to a melanoma in the lumbosacral area. [French] Syndrome queue-de-cheval resultant d'un melanome en region lombosacree. Pratique Vet Equine 2003;35:39–48.

47. Cudmore LA, Groenendyk JC, Hodge P, et al. Pyogranulomatous lesion causing neurological signs localised to the sacral region in a horse. Aust Vet J 2012;90:392–4.

48. Holt PE, Pearson H. Urolithiasis in the horse - a review of thirteen cases. Equine Vet J 1984;16:31–4.

49. Holt P, Mair TS. Ten cases of bladder paralysis associated with sabulous urolithiasis in horses. Vet Rec 1990;127:108–10.

50. Keen JA, Pirie RS. Urinary incontinence associated with sabulous urolithiasis: a series of 4 cases. Equine Vet Educ 2006;18:11–6.

51. Rendle DI, Durham AE, Hughes KJ, et al. Long-term management of sabulous cystitis in five horses. Vet Rec 2008;162:783–8.

52. Fonteque JH, Granella MCS, Souza AF, et al. Chronic renal failure in equine due to ascending pyelonephritis predisposed by cauda equina syndrome: case report. Arquivo Brasileiro de Medicina Veterinaria e Zootecnia 2018;70:347–52.

53. Onmaz AC, Atalan G, Pavaloiu AN, et al. A case report: recurrent cystitis in a mare. Kafkas Universitesi Veteriner Fakultesi Dergisi 2013;19(Suppl A):A203–6.

54. Paul-Jeanjean S. Post-partum disorders in mares. [French] Les affections du post-partum chez la jument. Pratique Vet Equine 2010;42:55–64.

55. Schumacher J, Brink P. Repair of an incompetent urethral sphincter in a mare. Vet Surg 2011;40:93–6.

56. Gehlen H, Klug E. Urinary incontinence in the mare due to iatrogenic trauma. Equine Vet Educ 2001;13:183–6.

57. Aleman M, Nieto JE, Higgins JK. Ulcerative cystitis associated with phenylbutazone administration in two horses. J Am Vet Med Assoc 2011;239:499–503.

58. Madison JB. Estrogen-responsive urinary incontinence in an aged pony mare. Compend Contin Educ Pract Vet 1984;6:S390.

59. Watson ED, McGorum BC, Keeling N, et al. Oestrogen-responsive urinary incontinence in two mares. Equine Vet Educ 1997;9:81–4.

60. Morgan RA, Malalana F, McGowan CM. Nephrogenic diabetes insipidus in a 14-year-old gelding. N Z Vet J 2012;60:254–7.

61. Adams LG, Dollahite JW, Romane WM, et al. Cystitis and ataxia associated with sorghum ingestion by horses. J Am Vet Med Assoc 1969;155:518–24.
62. Van Kampen AR. Sudan grass and sorghum poisoning of horses: a possible lathyrogenic disease. J Am Vet Med Assoc 1970;156:629–30.
63. Knight PR. Equine cystitis and ataxia associated with grazing pastures dominated by sorghum species. Aust Vet J 1968;44:257.

Polyuria and Polydipsia in Horses

Emily A. Barrell, DVM, MSc

KEYWORDS

- Polyuria • Polydipsia • Diabetes • Psychogenic • PPID • Urine • Vasopressin
- ADH

KEY POINTS

- Polyuria and polydipsia are rare clinical signs with numerous potential causes; in horses, the most common causes of PU/PD are chronic kidney disease, pituitary pars intermedia dysfunction (PPID), and psychogenic polydipsia with secondary polyuria.
- All investigations into polyuria and polydipsia should begin with history, physical examination, urine specific gravity, and chemistry profile.
- Important iatrogenic causes of polyuria include overhydration via fluid therapy and administration of drugs that either act directly on the kidney or incite acute or chronic renal failure with use.
- Psychogenic polydipsia must be distinguished from diabetes insipidus by means of a water deprivation test or, if long-standing with resultant medullary washout, modified water deprivation test.

INTRODUCTION

Polyuria (PU), defined as an increased volume of urine, is a rare, but significant, clinical manifestation of a wide variety of diseases (**Box 1**). Polydipsia (PD), or excessive thirst and fluid intake, is the natural companion to PU because these two clinical signs nearly always occur together. However, distinguishing which clinical sign is primary is an important task for the practitioner. That said, although primary PD with resultant PU does occur, primary PU with secondary PD is more likely in most cases.[1] As such, this article primarily focuses on PU, with a brief mention of primary, psychogenic PD.

The maintenance fluid requirement for a healthy, adult horse is ~50 to 60 mL/kg body weight (BW)/day, although this number can vary greatly based on environmental factors, exercise, pregnancy status, illness, and more.[2] Urine production in healthy, adult horses is 15 to 30 mL/kg BW/d, or approximately 10 to 15 L per day for an average, 500-kg horse.[1] The volume of urine produced depends on water consumption but is also the result of numerous environmental and physiologic factors, diet, gut

Department of Veterinary Population Medicine, University of Minnesota College of Veterinary Medicine, 1365 Gortner Avenue, VPM 225, Saint Paul, MN 55108, USA
E-mail address: ebarrell@umn.edu

Vet Clin Equine 38 (2022) 95–108
https://doi.org/10.1016/j.cveq.2021.11.007
0749-0739/22/© 2021 Elsevier Inc. All rights reserved.

> **Box 1**
> **Causes of polyuria in the horse.**
>
> Endocrine
>   Diabetes Insipidus (DI)
>   Central DI
>   Nephrogenic DI
>   Diabetes Mellitus (DM)
>   Pituitary Pars Intermedia Dysfunction (PPID)*
>
> Iatrogenic
>   Corticosteroids
>   Prednisolone, dexamethasone, triamcinolone, methylprednisolone, etc.
>   α-2 adrenergic receptor agonists
>   Xylazine, detomidine, dexmedetomidine
>   Diuretics
>   Fluid therapy
>   Excessive dietary salt
>   Nephrotoxic drugs
>   Gentamicin, oxytetracycline, polymyxin B, amphotericin B, etc.
>
> Psychogenic
>   Primary*
>   With or without medullary washout
>   Salt consumption
>   Hepatic encephalopathy
>
> Renal
>   Postobstructive diuresis
>   Chronic renal disease*
>   Acute kidney injury
>   Neoplasia
>
> Infectious
>   Peritonitis
>   Pyelonephritis
>   Pyometra
>   Renal helminth infection
>
> Toxic
>   *Datura stramonium* (thorn apple)#
>   Organophosphate
>   Cantharidin
>   Vitamin D
>   Calcium
>
> Other
>   Chronic liver disease
>
> *Most common causes of PU/polydipsia in the horse.[38]
>
> #Not reported in the United States.
>
> *Adapted from* Barrell EA, Burton AJ. Alterations in urinary function. In: Smith BP, Van Metre DC, Pusterla N, editors. Large animal internal medicine. 6th edition. Saint Louis, Missouri: Elsevier; 2020, 172.

fill, and water losses via other routes (eg, feces, sweat). Notably, because of their milk diet and higher total body water, daily maintenance fluid requirements for neonatal foals are much higher at ~250 mL/kg BW/d and normal foals will produce urine volumes of up to 148 mL/kg BW/d.[2]

An adult horse with PD will have a daily fluid intake in excess of 100 mL/kg BW/d, and horses with PU will often have urine production in excess of 50 mL/kg BW/d.[2] Once it has been determined that the patient meets one or both of these criteria, investigation into the cause of PU and/or PD begins. A thorough history of both the horse and the farm should be obtained, with special attention given to previous illness and medication history, housing and environmental conditions, diet, and feeding regimen. Examination of the horse from a distance allows for assessment of behavior, posture, gait, and urination. Physical examination of the patient should be routine and complete, with extra attention paid to mentation, body condition, oral cavity, mucous membranes, and external genitalia.

Diagnostics can be performed in a stepwise manner, but all investigations of PU should start with, at minimum, a chemistry profile and urine collection for evaluation for the presence of azotemia, hyperglycemia, and electrolyte derangements, and measurement of urine specific gravity (USG), respectively (**Fig. 1**). USG is the most valuable point-of-care test for evaluating renal concentrating ability. USG is used to compare the density of urine with that of water; water has a specific gravity of 1.000. If serum electrolytes and osmolarity are in the normal range, a USG of less than 1.008 is considered hyposthenuric and USG of 1.008 to 1.014 would be

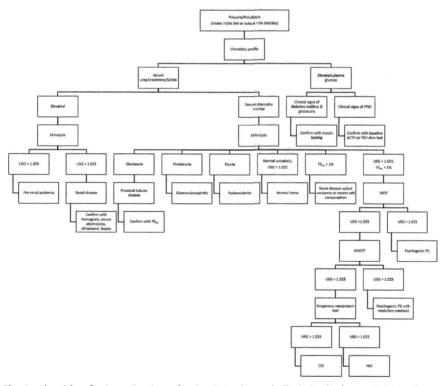

Fig. 1. Algorithm for investigation of polyuria and/or polydipsia in the horse. ACTH, adrenocorticotropic hormone; CDI, central diabetes insipidus; FE_{Na}, fractional excretion of sodium; MWDT, modified water deprivation test; NDI, nephrogenic diabetes insipidus; PPID, pituitary pars intermedia dysfunction; SDMA, symmetric dimethylarginine; TRH, thyrotropin-releasing hormone; WDT, water deprivation test. (*Adapted from* Knottenbelt DC. Polyuria-polydipsia in the horse. Equine Vet Educ. 2000;12:184

isosthenuric (same or similar tonicity as plasma). Under conditions of extreme dehydration, healthy adult kidneys can concentrate urine to at least a USG of 1.055, which is equivalent to an osmolality of nearly 2000 mOsmol/kg.[3] Foals, due to their large consumption of milk, commonly have hyposthenuric urine; healthy adult horses rarely have hyposthenuric urine. USG should always be evaluated in light of hydration status, treatments such as fluids and diuretics, and serum chemistry values. Urine multisticks do not provide an accurate measure of USG so a refractometer should always be used for this purpose.

Additional blood work such as a hemogram; measurement of symmetric dimethylarginine (SDMA), adrenocorticotropic hormone (ACTH), insulin, or bile acids; or performance of a thyrotropin-releasing hormone (TRH) response test may be the necessary next steps. Urinalysis and fractional clearance of sodium or other solutes may be useful for identifying early renal disease, whereas water deprivation test (WDT) and modified water deprivation test (MWDT) will help the practitioner distinguish psychogenic PD from diabetes insipidus (DI). More advanced testing such as renal ultrasonography, vasopressin response test, and renal biopsy are occasionally needed to diagnosis the underlying cause of PU.

THIRST, WATER CONSUMPTION, AND URINE PRODUCTION IN NORMAL HORSES

Healthy horses drink approximately 25 to 70 mL of water/kg BW/d, and a 500-kg, healthy horse may drink, on average, approximately 50 L or 13 gallons of water each day.[4,5] This amount will vary greatly depending on environmental and physiologic circumstances (eg, lactation, activity, diet, time of day). Another variable affecting amount of water consumed daily is whether the horse is pastured or stalled, and bolus feeding can have a profound effect on increasing water consumption in horses. An increase in water consumption following bolus feeding is presumably an attempt to correct extracellular dehydration caused by water moving from the extracellular fluid compartment into the hypertonic ingesta in the gastrointestinal tract.[6] Conversely, feed deprivation and decreased amount of ingesta in the intestinal tract reduces voluntary water consumption in horses.[6] Management practices should accommodate these drinking patterns of horses by providing water ad libitum in association with meals.[7] The temperature, tonicity, and quality of water may also affect water consumption, and horses will generally drink more water from buckets than automatic water bowls.[8]

Thirst and water consumption are controlled by two predominant physiologic mechanisms: the need to maintain plasma volume and serum osmolality. Of the two, a minor increase in serum osmolality is a more sensitive stimulus for thirst than is a decrease in plasma volume or total body water. The research of Dr. Katherine Houpt, a pioneer in the area of equine behavioral physiology, discovered that ponies had an increase in thirst with a 3% increase in osmolality, whereas a 6% decrease in plasma volume was needed to increase thirst in the same ponies.[9] Increased osmolality of blood and decreased plasma volume also cause a rapid release of antidiuretic hormone (ADH) into circulation, and it might be possible that sufficiently high ADH concentrations could directly stimulate thirst. Increased serum levels of angiotensin II are also known to directly increase thirst in many species.[10,11] Another poorly understood mechanism for increasing thirst is an abnormal dryness of the mouth, pharynx, and esophagus. Although unproven, this increase in thirst may be associated with visceral osmoreceptors and the autonomic nervous system, which activate thirst centers in the brain. Amazingly, in some species, this stimulus will cause the animal to quickly drink the amount of water they need to correct osmolar or fluid deficits, and they then stop drinking well before the water is absorbed into plasma and increased plasma osmolarity and intravascular volume deficits are corrected. Similar findings have been reported when horses deprived of food and water for 72 hours during periods of high environmental temperatures were allowed to drink.[10,12]

In healthy animals, approximately 99% of the water in the glomerular filtrate is resorbed as it flows through the nephron tubular system. Water resorption in the renal tubules occurs by the following mechanisms: passive reabsorption in segments of the nephron that have aquaporin proteins on the tubular epithelium, cotransport following the active ion transport in certain segments of the tubule, and in association with neuroendocrine influences, which occur mostly in the distal tubules.[13] Reabsorbed water from renal tubules is returned to circulation by the peritubular and vasa recta capillaries. The proximal tubules are responsible for 70% of the water resorption, the thin descending loop of Henle 15%, and the collecting tubules approximately 15%. Other parts of the tubules are relatively impermeable to water because they have little aquaporin expression. Both sodium and chloride are reabsorbed throughout the ascending loop of Henle and the distal convoluted tubule with little water resorbed.[14] Finally, the resorption of water is highly variable in the distal nephron (medullary collecting ducts) and depends on plasma volume and tonicity and the related neurohormonal influences (eg, ADH, aldosterone, atrial natriuretic peptide).[13]

POLYURIA CAUSED BY CHRONIC RENAL FAILURE

Unlike humans where hypertension and diabetes mellitus (DM) are the most common causes of chronic renal failure (CRF) and end-stage renal disease, nephrotoxic drugs, toxins, myopathy, and anomalies of development are the more likely causes of CRF in horses.[15,16] Although CRF has many different causes, and regardless of whether the inciting disease was primarily glomerular or tubulointerstitial in origin, the end result is always the same: progressive loss of functional nephrons.[17] In the initial stages of CRF, when nephrons are lost, the kidneys attempt to adapt via an increase in blood flow and glomerular filtration rate (GFR), which results in increased urine output (PU) by the remaining, functional nephrons.[15] This increase in GFR and blood flow is thought to be made possible by hypertrophy of the remaining nephrons, decreased vascular resistance, and decreased tubular reabsorption.[15] Eventually, however, these adaptations damage the kidneys further; increased pressure and stretch on the glomeruli lead to injury and sclerosis of small vessels and subsequent destruction of the glomerular architecture.[15] In response, the kidney undergoes further adaptive changes, and the process repeats itself until end-stage renal disease occurs.[15]

Although PU and loss of the ability to concentrate urine are relatively common signs of CRF, these sometimes go unnoticed by owners because the PU associated with CRF is moderate in volume when compared with the PU of DI or psychogenic PD. This is especially true if an animal is housed with other horses or is on pasture, making it hard to know how much urine an individual horse is producing.[16,17] Additional clinical signs are somewhat dependent on the stage of CRF, but often include weight loss, ventral edema, rough or dull hair coat, decreased appetite, dental tartar and oral ulcers, melena, and poor performance.[16]

Diagnosis of CRF can be simple in advanced stages but may require more advanced testing in early stages. To begin, the practitioner should collect urine and blood for hemogram, chemistry profile, and urinalysis. Abnormalities on blood work will vary to some degree, and it is worth noting that at least 65% of nephrons must become nonfunctional before elevations in these routinely used kidney function biomarkers will be detected.[16] In some cases, nephron loss approaches 75% or more before changes in serum creatinine and blood urea nitrogen (BUN) are detectable.[18] Electrolyte abnormalities can include hyperkalemia, hyponatremia, hypochloremia, hypercalcemia, hypomagnesemia, and normal to decreased phosphorous. Metabolic acidosis will occur in end-stage CRF. Anemia secondary to decreased production of erythropoietin by the kidneys will often be detected on hemogram.

In cases of early CRF, when there are only mild changes in GFR, azotemia and iso-sthenuria are not consistently present, so additional, more sensitive diagnostics are necessary. Fractional excretion of electrolytes, namely sodium, can provide useful information about tubule function in patients suspected to have early or mild CRF who may have normal creatinine and BUN concentrations and are still able to concentrate urine.[2,19] To perform this test, salt and fluid intake must be normal and the patient must not have received diuretics or intravenous (IV) or oral fluids. Urine and blood are collected simultaneously, and creatinine and sodium levels are measured in each sample. The fractional clearance (Fc %) is then determined by use of a formula, such as shown below for sodium

$$Fc_{Na}(\%) = \frac{[Na_u]}{[Na_p]} \times \frac{[Cr_p]}{[Cr_u]} \times 100$$

where Na_u is the urine sodium concentration, Na_p is the plasma sodium concentration, Cr_u is the urine creatinine concentration, and Cr_p is the plasma creatinine concentration. Normal values for fractional excretion of sodium in horses are 1% or less; values greater than this are supportive of primary renal tubular disease.[19]

In addition to fractional excretion, the urine protein to urine creatinine ratio (UP:UC) can be useful in detecting changes in GFR and damage. Normal horses will have ratios < 0.5, whereas large amounts of protein in the urine, and subsequent UP:UC ratios of > 0.5, are generally due to glomerular, rather than tubular, disease.

Measurement of SDMA is routinely used in human and small animal medicine as a more sensitive diagnostic for detecting kidney damage, and a validated test now exists for horses. This endogenous form of arginine is released into circulation during normal protein catabolism, and 90% of SDMA is excreted by the kidneys into urine in an unchanged form.[20] As such, this metabolite accumulates with prerenal or renal dysfunction and few nonrenal factors affect SDMA concentrations, making this a relatively specific assessment. Normal values have been established for both healthy adults and foals, and comparison of SDMA values between healthy animals and those with elevated creatinine and/or acute kidney injury have been performed.[20–23] An increased SDMA concentration was shown to correspond with disease severity, and SDMA was able to correctly distinguish between healthy and ill horses.[20]

Additional diagnostics, such as transabdominal or rectal renal ultrasonography or, in rare cases, renal biopsy, may be necessary to arrive at a final diagnosis of CRF.

POSTOBSTRUCTIVE DISEASE

Complete urinary obstruction is uncommon in horses, but the postobstructive PU that occurs after resolution of an obstruction can be marked.[17] Possible causes for increased volume of urine following relief of an obstruction include the elimination of retained solutes, such as urea, with secondary water diuresis, a blunted response to ADH, and/or defective sodium reabsorption. Decreased expression of aquaporins in the distal tubules and collecting ducts can last for up to 2 weeks.[17] Increased expression and activation of prostaglandin and nitric oxide receptors such as P2Y, EP1, and EP3 and subsequent release of inflammatory mediators may also contribute to postobstructive PU.[17] In addition to transient PU following relief of complete obstruction, long-term impairment of the ability to concentrate urine can also occur. Mechanisms of this dysfunction include reduced aquaporin expression and marked downregulation of sodium and urea transporters.[17]

DIABETES INSIPIDUS

DI is a rare cause of PU in horses and occurs due to either a deficiency of vasopressin, termed central or neurogenic diabetes insipidus (CDI), or an insensitivity of the renal tubules to vasopressin, known as nephrogenic diabetes insipidus (NDI). In contrast to DM, which is characterized by insulin deficiency (type 1 DM) or insulin resistance (type 2 DM), horses with DI will have normal blood glucose levels and no glucosuria. Clinical signs will include enormous volumes of dilute urine due to decreased water absorption by the renal tubules, and DI must often be distinguished from psychogenic PD/PU because the two diseases manifest in similar ways.

To diagnose DI, psychogenic PU/PD must first be ruled out by means of a WDT; an additional step of MWDT may also be necessary. The WDT is only indicated in horses with hyposthenuric urine (<1.008). WDT should not be performed in horses that are dehydrated or azotemic because withholding of water will only exacerbate these conditions. It is worth noting that horses with loss of 65% or less renal function may not be azotemic and may still be able to concentrate urine, but WDT would be detrimental to these patients. These horses would have some increase in serum creatinine and urea nitrogen levels, but values might still be in the normal reference range. In these cases, fractional excretion and/or urine protein to urine creatinine ratio would be useful in evaluating renal tubule function and glomerular function, respectively. Owing to these risks, all other causes of PU should be ruled out before considering this test. In healthy animals, a normal response to water withdrawal is a rapid increase in plasma osmolality leading to vasopressin release and subsequent urine concentration; normal horses will have a USG of 1.040–1.054 after 48 hours of deprivation.[24]

The WDT begins by collecting baseline blood and urine samples. Next, the bladder is emptied manually via catheterization, the horse is weighed, and water is removed. BW and USG are measured at least every 6 to 12 hours, and other indicators of hydration, such as packed cell volume (PCV), total solids, mucous membrane examination, heart rate, skin tent, and others, are monitored more frequently. The test is stopped when (1) the target USG is reached within 24 hours, (2) the horse loses 5% or more of its initial BW, or (3) evidence of dehydration or azotemia is identified.[24] In a horse with uncomplicated psychogenic PD, the USG will be 1.025 or higher at the conclusion of the test. A persistently dilute urine of USG 1.008 or less indicates either CDI or NDI. A USG of greater than 1.008 but less than 1.020 can occur with partial CDI, or with long-standing psychogenic PD that has resulted in medullary washout. In these cases, a MWDT is required. Once the horse has recovered from the initial WDT and is fully rehydrated, water is restricted to 40 mL/kg/d for 3 to 4 days.[24] Hydration status and USG are closely monitored, and a horse with medullary washout and psychogenic PD should be able to form concentrated urine within 72 to 96 hours of initiation of the test. Horses that have a persistently isosthenuric USG following a modified WDT are suspected to have CDI.

Testing to distinguish CDI and NDI requires measurement of endogenous or administration of exogenous vasopressin. Measuring endogenous vasopressin during a WDT can help to distinguish the two diseases. Elevated vasopressin with dilute urine indicates an inability of the kidneys to appropriately respond to vasopressin and would indicate NDI. A low or relatively low plasma vasopressin concentration given the plasma osmolality, along with dilute urine, during a WDT would support a diagnosis of CDI. However, because of the inherent instability of this hormone and because it can be challenging to find a laboratory capable of measuring plasma vasopressin, an alternative method of distinguishing CDI from NDI is often necessary.

The exogenous vasopressin test is used to assess the renal tubules' ability to appropriately respond to a synthetic vasopressin. One option for performing this test is aqueous synthetic vasopressin. This solution can be given at a dose of 0.25 to 0.5 U/kg intramuscularly or as an infusion (5 U diluted in 1 L 5% dextrose [2.5 mU/kg] administered over 60 minutes).[24] With CDI, USG should increase to 1.020 or more within 90 minutes; lack of urine concentration over the same period would indicate NDI.[24] Desmopressin acetate (DDAVP) solution is an alternative to aqueous synthetic vasopressin. DDAVP given at a dose of 0.05 μg/kg IV should result in a USG increase to 1.025 or higher within 2 hours for CDI, whereas no response would support NDI if psychogenic PD with medullary washout has been ruled out.

Potential treatment of DI is limited to CDI; case reports of NDI describe only dietary management and salt and water limitation as means of managing horses with NDI.[25–27] Although several different pharmaceuticals have been proposed for the treatment of CDI in horses, only use of vasopressin in the form of desmopressin has been documented.[28–30] A 2010 report by Kranenburg and colleagues[29] described the successful use of desmopressin acetate hydrate eye drops in a 10-day-old Friesian colt with congenital CDI. While in hospital, use of a human formulation of nasal drops resulted in urine concentration within 4 hours of initial administration. In a more recent case report by Durie and van Galen,[30] a 4-year-old, Warmblood, gelding with excessive water consumption of 5× to 6.5× maintenance requirements and hyposthenuric urine was diagnosed with CDI following WDT and MWDT. Treatment included administration of desmopressin in the form of a human nasal spray, administered first via intraocular route and then as a subcutaneous injection. Five years of follow-up revealed that the horse was doing well and required only minor dosage adjustments as he aged and gained weight.[30]

Because of the potential hereditary component to DI, as evidenced by the case report by Schott and colleagues[26] of 2 full sibling Thoroughbred colts with NDI, recommending against breeding may be advisable.

DIABETES MELLITUS

In contrast to the ADH abnormalities associated with DI, DM is characterized by insulin deficiency (type 1 DM) due to destruction of β pancreatic cells, or insulin resistance (type 2 DM). Both classic type 1 and type 2 DM are infrequently reported in the equine literature. PU, PD, and weight loss are common presenting complaints for horses with type 2 DM, and most case reports document horses of advanced age.[31] Affected horses will have elevated blood glucose and many will have glucosuria, of which the latter results in an osmotic diuresis and subsequent PU.[32] Hypertriglyceridemia, sometimes with the presence of gross lipemia, may also be present.[32] Insulin levels can be low, normal, or elevated.

Many, but not all, horses with type 2 DM will be concurrently diagnosed with pituitary pars intermedia dysfunction (PPID), with the insulin resistance of the PPID suggested as the mechanism for hyperglycemia and osmotic diuresis seen in horses with type 2 DM.

Although resting insulin concentration, oral and IV glucose tolerance tests, IV insulin tolerance test, and response to treatment are relatively easy to perform, specific (but arguably more technically challenging) tests for insulin sensitivity and β pancreatic cell function may be more appropriate. More specific tests of β cell function and insulin sensitivity include the hyperinsulinemic-euglycemic clamp and hyperglycemic clamp techniques, as well as the insulin-modified frequently sampled IV glucose tolerance test (I-FSIGT$_{MM}$).[31]

Treatment of DM has been attempted and described in the literature, although with limited success due to the cost, adverse effects, and/or questionable efficacy of medications such as insulin, metformin, and so forth. Treatment of type 1 DM in a pony with protamine zinc insulin was reportedly successful, but even high doses of insulin in some cases of type 2 DM have been unsuccessful.[32] Because of the frequent link between DM and PPID, pergolide is a reasonable treatment choice, especially in horses with clinical signs or blood work (baseline ACTH, TRH stimulation test) that support underlying PPID as a cause for DM. Durham and colleagues[31] described 3 cases of DM in aged Warmbloods; diagnosis was made by I-FSIGT testing. Treatments included metformin, oral glibenclamide, dietary modification, and/or pergolide, and responses were fair to moderate, depending on the case.[31] Baseline ACTH concentration was elevated in one of the 3 horses, supportive of PPID as a cause for the insulin resistance. However, this was not the case for the other 2 horses.

CUSHING DISEASE

The incidence of PU in horses with PPID is estimated to be around 33%, although values are highly variable with some studies reporting 0% incidence of PU as a reported clinical sign of PPID and others reporting 76% incidence of PU.[33–35] The mechanism by which PPID induces PU has not been thoroughly researched, but several proposed theories exist in both small animal and equine medicine. First, it is postulated that the excessive ACTH action on the adrenal cortex with subsequent hypercortisolemia is a driving factor for the PU of PPID.[2] Elevated cortisol in the blood directly increases glucose formation and promotes insulin resistance, resulting in hyperglycemia, glucosuria, and osmotic diuresis. Although this is frequently the mechanism cited in small animal medicine to explain the partial DM that occurs with hyperadrenocorticism, little evidence exists to support this in either canine or equine medicine.[36] In a case report of horses with PPID, only 1 of 5 had glucosuria.[33]

Another possible explanation for PU that occurs with PPID is that growth of the pars intermedia directly compresses the posterior pituitary and hypothalamic nuclei, which are the sites of vasopressin storage and release. Physical impingement negatively affecting vasopressin secretion would result in partial CDI and, without vasopressin to act on the renal tubule cells and collecting ducts, concentration of urine would not be possible.[2] However, some horses with PPID are able to concentrate their urine in the face of a WDT.

It is also possible that the excess cortisol produced in cases of PPID antagonizes the action of vasopressin in the renal collect ducts.[2] Without vasopressin, the aquaporin channels along the apical membrane of the principal cells would be decreased in number or absent, resulting in an inability to move water from the tubular fluid back into circulation and, ultimately, an inability to concentrate urine. Unfortunately, experimental evidence for this proposed mechanism is lacking.

Last, the hirsutism that occurs with PPID may lead to increased sweating and fluid loss, prompting increased thirst.[36]

Ultimately, it is likely that some combination of these mechanisms and, potentially, others are responsible for the PU observed in some cases of PPID.

FLUID THERAPY AS A CAUSE OF POLYURIA

One of the most common iatrogenic causes of PU in equine patients is overhydration via IV fluid therapy, and both water and solute diuresis can be underlying mechanisms for the increased volume of urine produced. Commercial solutions used for fluid therapy are often too rich in sodium. Horses on maintenance IV fluids can receive 10× their normal daily intake of sodium, which induces diuresis and electrolyte movement.[6] This increase in plasma sodium can also result in sodium secretion into the GI tract, quadrupling sodium output in feces and decreasing plasma sodium concentration in water-deprived horses, such as those off feed for colic or other reasons, worsening dehydration that already exists.[6] Sodium is lost in the urine when using commercial solutions, and there are also clinically significant loses of potassium, calcium, and magnesium.[37] Additional adverse effects of overhydration with IV fluid therapy include rebound dehydration, edema, impaired lymphatic drainage, poorer anesthetic recovery, and increased cost to the client.[6,38]

Because maintenance fluid requirements were derived from fed horses and horses naturally drink less water when they are not eating, it has been proposed that horses off feed should have lower requirements.[6] Furthermore, 30% to 55% of daily water loss is via the feces, and horses that defecate less due to fasting, ileus, obstruction, or decreased feed intake lose less water.[6] Based on studies reporting feed deprivation reducing water consumption to ~16% of fed values, it has been recommended that horses off feed may need only ~10 mL/kg/d, as opposed to more standard suggestions of 50 to 60 mL/kg/d as a maintenance requirement.[6] Advantages of reducing the daily amount of fluids for a horse off feed include reduced volumes and lower cost, as well as avoidance of overhydration and electrolyte derangements.[6]

Rather than using a standard maintenance rate, evaluation of the effectiveness of fluid therapy should be performed regularly to titrate treatment doses to the individual patient. In general, when monitoring for changes in hydration status, trends are more useful than single or infrequent values or observations. Careful physical examination and monitoring that includes evaluation of mucous membrane color, capillary refill time, eye position, skin-tent duration, pulse character, extremity temperature, speed of jugular distention when the vein is manually occluded, and heart rate all give valuable information to the practitioner when making decisions about fluid requirements and rates. Serial measurements of BW, packed cell volume, and total solids can be useful to track improvements over time. Blood lactate can provide additional information about tissue perfusion, but care should be taken when interpreting because values can be normal despite significant perfusion deficits to individual tissues; again, trends over time can improve the value of this test.[39]

Monitoring of urine production and USG can and should be used to guide treatment decisions concerning fluid therapy. Hypovolemia and dehydration should result in concentrated urine (USG > 1.035), whereas isosthenuria would be expected with adequate resuscitation.[39] Hyposthenuria should not be the goal of fluid therapy. It is worth noting that some diseases, such as DI, may result in dilute urine (<1.008) in the face of hypovolemia, and care must be taken to prevent incorrect classification of these animals as adequately hydrated or overhydrated. Other hemodynamic parameters, such as central venous pressure, blood pressure, colloid oncotic pressure, and gastric tonometry, have all been used to evaluate the effectiveness of fluid therapy, although equipment and skill requirements result in infrequent usage outside of academic or research settings.[39]

OTHER CAUSES OF POLYURIA

In addition to IV fluids, drugs such as diuretics, sedatives, and corticosteroids can all be iatrogenic causes of PU in horses. Although various classes of diuretics have different mechanisms of action, all ultimately increase the rate and volume of urine output. Equine practitioners use alpha-2 adrenergic receptor agonists, such as xylazine and detomidine, daily, and PU is a known side effect following administration of these sedatives. Glucocorticoids such as prednisolone, dexamethasone, methylprednisolone, triamcinolone, naquasone, and others are known to cause PU in horses, although the exact mechanism by which this occurs is not known. Other drugs cause PU not by direct effects but by inciting acute or chronic injury to the kidneys. Aminoglycosides, oxytetracycline, nonsteroidal anti-inflammatories, polymyxin B, amphotericin B, imidocarb dipropionate, and bisphosphonates are all potentially nephrotoxic and have documented and/or anecdotal reports of renal disease following their use.[40]

Additional diseases associated with PU, either primarily via water or solute diuresis or secondarily via kidney injury, include but are not limited to liver failure, neoplasia, toxicities, inflammatory conditions, and parasitism (see **Box 1**).

PSYCHOGENIC POLYDIPSIA

The condition of primary or psychogenic PD is one of the most common causes of PD and subsequent PU in the horse.[1,36] Diet, management, and housing have all been implicated as factors contributing to the development of psychogenic PD. Sometimes considered a vice, psychogenic PD can be seen in horses housed in stalls; other behavioral abnormalities such as chewing on doors or eating bedding may also be observed.[1] Stressors such as changes in housing, management, and environment have also been reported to incite psychogenic PD.[1] Dietary factors such as high dry matter intake or compulsive salt consumption may lead to excessive water consumption. In one case report, a yearling Paint filly was presented for PU, a stiff gait, and muscle fasciculations; USG was 1.006 on presentation.[41] A 20-h WDT resulted in adequate concentration, ruling out CDI and NDI. Closer observation revealed that the filly consumed more salt than the other horses on the property, and water limitation and salt deprivation resolved all clinical signs.[41]

Horses with psychogenic PD will produce copious volumes of urine, much more so than those with PPID or CRF.[1] Owners often report that stalls or paddocks are soaking wet, and the horse drinks much more than others on the same property. Urine will be dilute at USG 1.005 or less, but these animals are not azotemic and usually are in good body condition. Results of a WDT will depend on the duration of the PD. Horses with uncomplicated, short-term PD will respond favorably to WDT and will be able to concentrate their urine. Those with long-standing PD are likely to have "medullary washout" and will require a MWDT to concentrate urine. Medullary washout following prolonged PU/PD occurs when the normal osmotic gradient that exists between the renal tubule lumen and the renal interstitium is lost, resulting in dilute urine.[42]

Managing psychogenic PD requires knowledge of the underlying cause. Management changes to reduce boredom can include increasing exercise and/or turnout. Reducing stressors in the environment may require housing the horse with an amenable companion, transitioning from stall housing to pasture housing, or moving the horse to a quieter portion of the property. Dietary considerations such as increasing the time a horse spends eating, either by using a slow-feed net or implementing small, frequent meals; supplementing electrolytes; or limiting water intake may all be beneficial on a case-by-case basis. In the rare cases of pathologic salt consumption, reducing or eliminating access to salt may be necessary, although the owner must be mindful of sweating due to exercise and the risk of salt loss.

DISCLOSURE

The author has nothing to disclose.

REFERENCES

1. Knottenbelt DC. Polyuria-polydipsia in the horse. Equine Vet Educ 2000;12: 179–86.
2. Hines M. Clinical approach to commonly encountered problems. In: Reed SM, Bayly WM, Sellon DC, editors. Equine internal medicine. 4th Edition. St. Louis, Missouri: Elsevier; 2018. p. 232–310.
3. Rumbaugh GE, Carlson GP, Harrold D. Urinary production in the healthy horse and in horses deprived of feed and water. Am J Vet Res 1982;43:735–7.
4. Lewis LD. Water, energy, protein, carbohydrates, and fats for horses. In: Feeding and care of the horse. 2nd Edition. Ames, Iowa: Lippincott Williams & Wilkins; 1996. p. 3.
5. National Research Council (U.S. Committee on Nutrient requirements of horses. Nutrient requirements of horses animal Nutrition Series. 6th Edition. Washington, (DC).: National Academies Press; 2007. p. 132.
6. Freeman DE, Mooney A, Giguere S, et al. Effect of feed deprivation on daily water consumption in healthy horses. Equine Vet J 2021;53:117–24.
7. Freeman DE. Effect of feed intake on water consumption in horses: relevance to maintenance fluid therapy. Front Vet Sci 2021;8:626081.
8. Nyman S, Dahlborn K. Effect of water supply method and flow rate on drinking behavior and fluid balance in horses. Physiol Behav 2001;73:1–8.
9. Sufit E, Houpt KA, Sweeting M. Physiological stimuli of thirst and drinking patterns in ponies. Equine Vet J 1985;17:12–6.
10. Houpt KA, Thornton SN, Allen WR. Vasopressin in dehydrated and rehydrated ponies. Physiol Behav 1989;45:659–61.
11. Fitzsimons JT. Angiotensin, thirst, and sodium appetite. Physiol Rev 1998;78: 583–686.
12. Carlson GP, Rumbaugh GE, Harrold D. Physiologic alterations in the horse produced by food and water deprivation during periods of high environmental temperatures. Am J Vet Res 1979;40:982–5.
13. Eaton DC, Pooler JP. Basic transport mechanisms; regulation of sodium and water excretion. In: Eaton DC, Pooler JP, editors. Vander's renal physiology. 9th Edition. New York, (NY): McGraw-Hill Education; 2018.
14. Nielsen S, Kwon TH, Christensen BM, et al. Physiology and pathophysiology of renal aquaporins. J Am Soc Nephrol 1999;10:647–63.
15. Hall JE, Hall ME. Diuretics and kidney diseases. In: Hall JE, Hall ME, editors. Guyton and Hall Textbook of medical physiology. 14th Edition. Philadelphia, PA: Elsevier; 2021. p. 421–35.
16. Divers TJ, Ollivett TL, McConachie Beasley E. Chronic renal failure. In: Smith BP, Van Metre DC, Pusterla N, editors. Large animal Internal medicine. 6th Edition. Saint Louis, Missouri: Elsevier; 2020. p. 963–7.
17. Nielsen S, Kwon T, Dimke H, et al. Aquaporin water channels in mammalian kidney. In: Alpern RJ, Moe OW, Caplan M, editors. Seldin and Giebisch's the kidney: physiology and Pathophysiology. 5th Edition. London: Elsevier; 2013. p. 1405–39.
18. Hokamp JA, Nabity MB. Renal biomarkers in domestic species. Vet Clin Pathol 2016;45:28–56.

19. Barrell EA, Burton AJ. Alterations in urinary function. In: Smith BP, Van Metre DC, Pusterla N, editors. Large animal Internal medicine. 6th Edition. Saint Louis, Missouri: Elsevier; 2020. p. 172–3.
20. Siwinska N, Zak A, Slowikowska M, et al. Serum symmetric dimethylarginine concentration in healthy horses and horses with acute kidney injury. BMC Vet Res 2020;16:396.
21. Schott HC, Gallant LR, Coyne M, et al. Symmetric dimethylarginine and creatinine concentrations in serum of healthy draft horses. J Vet Intern Med 2021;35:1147–54.
22. Bozorgmanesh R, Coyne M, Murphy R, et al. Equine neonatal symmetric dimethylarginine (SDMA): results of two pilot studies. J Vet Intern Med 2019;33:2440–1.
23. Bozorgmanesh R, Magdesian G, Offer K, et al. Equine neonatal symmetric dimethylarginine in sick neonates with hypercreatininemia. J Vet Emerg Crit Care 2019;29:S30.
24. McKenzie EC. Polyuria and polydipsia in horses. Vet Clin Equine 2007;23:641–53.
25. Brashier M. Polydipsia and polyuria in a weanling colt caused by nephrogenic diabetes insipidus. Vet Clin Equine 2006;22:219–27.
26. Schott HC, Bayly WM, Reed SM, et al. Nephrogenic diabetes insipidus in sibling colts. J Vet Intern Med 1993;7:68–72.
27. Morgan RA, Malalana F, McGowan CM. Nephrogenic diabetes insipidus in a 14-year-old gelding. N Z Vet J 2012;60:254–7.
28. Durham AE. Therapeutics for Equine Endocrine Disorders. Vet Clin Equine 2017;33:127–39.
29. Kranenburg LC, Thelen MHM, Westermann CM, et al. Use of desmopressin eye drops in the treatment of equine congenital central diabetes insipidus. Vet Rec 2010;167:790.
30. Durie I, van Galen G. Long-term hormone replacement treatment in a horse with central diabetes insipidus. J Vet Intern Med 2020;34:1013–7.
31. Durham AE, Hughes KJ, Cottle HJ, et al. Type 2 diabetes mellitus with pancreatic β cell dysfunction in 3 horses confirmed with minimal model analysis. Equine Vet J 2009;41:924–9.
32. Durham AE. Endocrine disease in aged horses. Vet Clin Equine 2016;32:301–15.
33. Schott HC. Pituitary pars intermedia dysfunction: equine Cushing's disease. Vet Clin Equine 2002;18:237–70.
34. Horn R, Bamford NJ, Afonso T, et al. Factors associated with survival, laminitis and insulin dysregulation in horses diagnosed with equine pituitary pars intermedia dysfunction. Equine Vet J 2019;51:440–5.
35. McGowan TW, Pinchbeck GP, McGowan CM. Prevalence, risk factors and clinical signs predictive for equine pituitary pars intermedia dysfunction in aged horses. Equine Vet J 2013;45:74–9.
36. Schott HC, Ollivett TL, Burton AJ. Polyuria and polydipsia. In: Smith BP, Van Metre DC, Pusterla N, editors. Large animal Internal medicine. 6th Edition. Saint Louis, Missouri: Elsevier; 2020. p. 977–9.
37. Lopes MA, Walker BL, White NA, et al. Treatments to promote colonic hydration: enteral fluid therapy versus intravenous fluid therapy and magnesium sulphate. Equine Vet J 2002;34:505–9.
38. Lester GD, Merritt AM, Kuck HV, et al. Systemic, renal, and colonic effects of intravenous and enteral rehydration in horses. J Vet Intern Med 2013;27:554–66.

39. Tennent-Brown B. Monitoring fluid therapy. In: Langdon Fielding C, Magdesian G, editors. Equine fluid therapy. 1st Edition. Ames, Iowa: John Wiley & Sons, Inc; 2015. p. 142–51.
40. Divers TJ, Burton AJ. Acute renal failure. In: Smith BP, Van Metre DC, Pusterla N, editors. Large animal Internal medicine. 6th Edition. Saint Louis, Missouri: Elsevier; 2020. p. 956–62.
41. Buntain BJ, Coffman JR. Polyuria and polydypsia in a horse induced by psychogenic salt consumption. Equine Vet J 1981;13(4):266–8.
42. Chew DJ, DiBartola SP, Schenck PA. Approach to polyuria and polydipsia. In: Chew DJ, Schench PA, DiBartola SP, editors. Canine and feline nephrology and urology. 2nd Edition. St. Louis, Missouri: Elsevier; 2011. p. 465–86.

Metabolic Disorders Associated with Renal Disease in Horses

Kathleen R. Mullen, DVM, MS

KEYWORDS

- Renal tubular acidosis • Calcinosis • Uremic encephalopathy
- Hyponatremic encephalopathy

KEY POINTS

- Renal tubular acidosis, a cause of hyperchloremic metabolic acidosis in horses, is usually responsive to alkali therapy although prolonged treatment and relapses are possible.
- Uremic encephalopathy is an uncommon sequela of renal failure in horses characterized by signs of cerebral cortical dysfunction.
- Foals with hyponatremic encephalopathy from acute kidney injury require careful monitoring and correction of the sodium deficit; it generally carries a favorable prognosis.
- Regulation of calcium and phosphorus homeostasis in the horse is unique, with important implications for renal disease.
- A syndrome of systemic calcinosis and calciphylaxis has been described in horses with myopathy, malaise, fever, and elevated calcium-phosphorus product; the etiology is unknown, and the prognosis is poor.

INTRODUCTION

The kidneys play a central role in acid–base regulation, filtration of uremic toxins, water and electrolyte balance, and calcium and phosphorus homeostasis. In disease states, these important roles are underscored. For example, renal tubular acidosis due to the failure of bicarbonate reabsorption in the renal proximal tubules or acid secretion in the collecting ducts results in hyperchloremic metabolic acidosis. Reduced excretion of uremic toxins in renal disease is thought to be the etiology of the complex pathogenesis of uremic encephalopathy and resulting histopathological lesions of diffuse central nervous system Alzheimer type II astrogliosis in horses. Retention of free water or excessive renal loss of sodium in foals with acute kidney injury can lead to the development of hyponatremic encephalopathy. Finally, renal disease can result in disorders of calcium and phosphorus homeostasis, for example, hypercalcemia of chronic renal disease. Likewise, disorders of calcium and phosphorus homeostasis, such as systemic calcinosis, can cause renal disease due to tubular and glomerular mineralization.

Littleton Equine Medical Center, 8025 South Santa Fe Drive, Littleton, CO 80120, USA
E-mail address: kmullen@littletonequine.com

Vet Clin Equine 38 (2022) 109–122
https://doi.org/10.1016/j.cveq.2021.11.008
0749-0739/22/© 2021 Elsevier Inc. All rights reserved.

In this article, the consequences of compromise of these various renal functions will be discussed with special emphasis on key factors for the recognition of clinical signs and diagnostic test results associated with each. Treatment options are presented along with prognosis to aid the practitioner in the management of these conditions.

DISCUSSION
Renal Tubular Acidosis Characterization and Pathophysiology

Renal tubular acidosis (RTA) occurs when the kidneys are unable to maintain normal acid–base homeostasis because of tubular defects in acid secretion or bicarbonate (HCO_3^-) reabsorption. RTA causes a normal anion gap hyperchloremic metabolic acidosis, whereby anion gap is defined as the difference between the number of cations (sodium and potassium) and anions (chloride and bicarbonate). The loss of serum bicarbonate results in a retention of chloride, so the anion gap remains normal.

In human medicine, 4 forms of RTA are recognized. Type 1 (distal) RTA is characterized by impaired acid secretion and evidence of potassium wasting. Defects in H^+ secretion by vacuolar H^+-ATPase or H^+/K^+-ATPase or increased H^+ permeability of the luminal membrane of the α-intercalated cells results in a net reduction in H^+ secretion (**Fig. 1**). Type 2 (proximal) RTA is caused by defects in the reabsorption of filtered HCO_3^- due to impaired HCO_3^- transport across the basolateral membrane or due to carbonic anhydrase inhibition.[1] Type 3 RTA is a rare form of the disease with features of both Type 1 and Type 2. Type 4 (hyperkalemic) RTA is caused by aldosterone deficiency or resistance, leading to decreased sodium (NA^+) absorption by principal cells in the collecting duct. This leads to a reduced transepithelial voltage resulting in decreased H^+ secretion by α -intercalated cells and K^+ secretion by principal cell.[1] (Palmer 2021). Type 4 RTA has not been described in horses.

RTA may be primary (inherited) or secondary (acquired). In humans, primary Type 1 RTA may be associated with autosomal mutations in the genes encoding for the vacuolar H^+-ATPase or basolateral $Cl^-/HCO3^-$ exchanger of the α-intercalated cells.[1] Secondary Type 1 RTA may result from medications including amphotericin B, ibuprofen, and lithium; it is also seen in association with systemic diseases.[1] Primary Type 2 RTA may be associated with mutations in the gene encoding the basolateral membrane $Na^+/HCO_3^-/CO_3^{2-}$ cotransporter (see **Fig. 1**) or acquired from the use of carbonic anhydrase inhibitors.[1]

Type 1 RTA may be associated with recurrent nephrolithiasis, nephrocalcinosis, and bone disease in humans, although this has not been observed in horses. H^+ retention also leads to decreases in renal calcium reabsorption and an increase in calcium release from bone, resulting in hypercalciuria.[1]

Type 2 RTA may occur as a single defect in HCO_3^- reabsorption, or more commonly in association with Fanconi syndrome that is characterized by widespread proximal tubule dysfunction that also includes the loss of glucose, phosphate, uric acid, amino acids, and low-molecular-weight proteins.[1] Human patients with Type 2 RTA and Fanconi Syndrome may develop osteomalacia due to chronic renal phosphate wasting. Osteopenia may result from acidosis-induced bone demineralization. Impaired conversion of 25(OH) vitamin D3 to 1,25 (OH)s vitamin D3 by 1α-hydroxylase in the proximal tubule may result in active hypovitaminosis D.[1] Note that horses do not rely on the renal activation of vitamin D, and hypovitaminosis D is an unlikely sequela in horses with Fanconi Syndrome.

Primary and secondary causes of Fanconi syndrome are observed in humans. Primary Fanconi syndrome is usually caused by a missense mutation in the sodium phosphate cotransporter in the proximal tubular apical membrane, although other

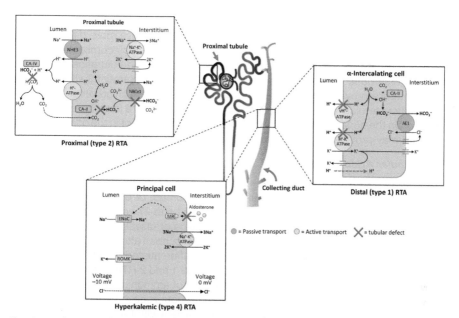

Fig. 1. A schematic diagram illustrating the underlying kidney tubule defects causing the different types of renal tubular acidosis (RTA). Distal (type 1) RTA is caused by either impaired hydrogen (H^+) secretion by vacuolar (v) H^+-ATPase or H^+/K^+-ATPase or increased H^+ permeability of luminal membrane by α-intercalated cells of the collecting duct, which leads to a reduction in net H^+ secretion. Proximal (type 2) RTA is caused by defects in bicarbonate (HCO_3^-) reabsorption in the proximal tubule, due to either impaired HCO_3^- transport across the basolateral membrane or inhibition of carbonic anhydrase (CA) activity. Hyperkalemic (type 4) RTA is caused by aldosterone deficiency or resistance, which leads to reduced Na^+ (sodium) reabsorption by principal cells of the collecting duct and decreased transepithelial voltage, leading to diminished H^+ secretion by α-intercalated cells and K^+ secretion by principal cells. Type 4 RTA has not been reported in horses. AE1 kidney anion exchanger, ENaC epithelial Na^+ channel, MR mineralocorticoid receptor, NHE3 Na^+/H^+ exchanger 3, ROMK apical membrane K^+ channel. (*From* Palmer BF, Kelepouris E, Clegg DJ. Renal Tubular Acidosis and Management Strategies: A Narrative Review. Adv Ther. 2021;38(2):949-968. https://doi.org/10.1007/s12325-020-01587-5; with permission.)

mutations have also recently been described.[2] Fanconi syndrome can also be associated with inherited systemic diseases. Among the secondary causes are acquired systemic diseases (amyloidosis, multiple myeloma, tubulo-interstitial nephritis), drugs (including some nucleotide reverse-transcriptase inhibitors, anticancer medications, anti-convulsants, antibiotics in particular aminoglycosides and outdated tetracycline, and DNA polymerase inhibitors), and heavy metals (lead, cadmium, and mercury). Most commonly Fanconi syndrome is a result of drug-induced nephrotoxicity.[2]

Classification of RTA in humans is based on symptoms, urine pH, serum HCO_3^- and potassium (K^+), and ancillary diagnostic tests including ammonium loading test, fractional excretion of HCO_3^-, HCO_3^- loading test, urinary K^+ concentration, fractional excretion of K^+, and serum aldosterone concentration. For example, patients with Type 1 RTA, tend to have a lower serum HCO_3^- (10–20 mEq/L) and higher urine pH > 5.3. Patients with Type 2 RTA may have higher serum HCO_3^- (16–20 mEq/L), lower urine pH < 5.5, and increased fractional excretion of HCO_3^- greater than 15%. In addition, patients with Type 2 RTA and Fanconi Syndrome may have other signs of proximal tubule dysfunction. Accurate diagnosis allows for optimal patient management and treatment.[1] Classification of RTA in horses can prove more difficult.

The mainstay of treatment in human medicine is alkali therapy combined with supplemental potassium in patients that are hypokalemic. Thiazide diuretics are used to enhance bicarbonate reabsorption in Type 2 RTA and supplemental vitamin D and phosphate are provided as needed in patients with Fanconi Syndrome.[2] In Type 4 RTA, corticosteroids, loop diuretics, and potassium binders are used to reduce hyperkalemia. On the horizon, are selective H^+ binding agents that act in the gastrointestinal tract and may provide an alternative to alkali therapy.[1]

Renal Tubular Acidosis in Horses

RTA is well described in horses.[3-15] Presenting complaints include anorexia, depression, weight loss, and poor performance. No sex, breed, or dietary predilection has been determined. Age at onset ranges from 6 months to 27 years. In a retrospective study of 16 cases, 10 had evidence of renal damage or disease.[3]

Type 1, 2, and mixed (Type 3) RTA[13] have been described although classification remains challenging, therefore, many cases are undifferentiated.[3] Ammonium chloride challenge can be used to distinguish between Type 1 and 2 RTA in horses. Normally, following administration per nasogastric intubation of ammonium chloride 0.1 g/kg of body weight, diluted in 6L water, urine acidification should occur. Inability to lower urine pH (<6.5) 2 to 4-hours postchallenge would be consistent with Type 1 RTA.[4,14] Additionally, when urine partial pressure of carbon dioxide, total carbon dioxide, and HCO_3^- concentrations are higher than blood concentrations, Type 2 RTA is suspected.[4]

Acquired Fanconi syndrome was diagnosed in two-Quarter horses with weight loss, mild metabolic acidosis, glucosuria, and euglycemia based on a semi-quantitative Fanconi screening test performed at the Metabolic Genetics Laboratory of the University of Pennsylvania.[7] Although not validated in horses, the results were compared with contemporary and historic equine controls and revealed aminoaciduria, lactic acidosis, and glucosuria in both cases.

Treatment of RTA in horses is primarily aimed at correcting metabolic acidosis regardless of the type of RTA. As horses with RTA commonly present dehydrated and azotemic, fluid therapy aimed at correcting hydration status is imperative. Horses with RTA are often anorectic and therefore may be hypokalemic at presentation, or they may develop hypokalemia during the correction of the metabolic acidosis as K^+ shifts into the intracellular space and H^+ move out. Providing oral potassium citrate rather than potassium chloride following initial intravenous fluid therapy is recommended.[4] Feeding forage once the patient is willing to eat will also help correct the hypokalemia. While individualized treatment plans are required for each case, a starting point is provided here (**Box 1**).

Response to treatment with intravenous sodium bicarbonate and potassium chloride is generally good, although protracted treatment with oral sodium bicarbonate may be required and relapses are possible, particularly in patients with underlying renal disease.[3] Long-term monitoring is indicated in patients requiring prolonged oral bicarbonate administration and in patients that have the recurrence of clinical signs associated with initial presentation. In the author's experience, relapses often follow management changes or inadvertent missed doses of bicarbonate in horses requiring long-term treatment.

Uremic Encephalopathy

Uremic encephalopathy (UE) is reported in humans and a variety of animal species including horses, cattle, goats, dogs, woodchucks, a coyote, and a rhesus

---

Box 1
Estimation of bicarbonate deficit and initial plan for the treatment of RTA in Horses

Estimation of HCO_3^- deficit $[mEq]$ = body weight $[kg] x$ volume of distribution x HCO_3^-

deficit $\left[mEq_{/L} \right]$

Volume of distribution = 0.3

HCO_3^- deficit $[mEq / L]$ = low end of HCO_3^- reference range $\left[mEq_{/L} \right]$ $--$ patients HCO_3^- $\left[mEq_{/L} \right]$

- Commercial injectable sodium bicarbonate is commonly available as a 5% or 8.5% solution.
- The 5% solution has 0.6 mEq/mL and the 8.4% solution has 1 mEq/mL HCO_3^-.
- To make an approximately isotonic solution, 1 L of 5% IV sodium bicarbonate can be diluted in 3L of sterile water. Alternatively, 150 mL of the 8.4% solution can be added to 1L of sterile water.
- One gram of oral sodium bicarbonate (baking soda) contains 12 mEq HCO_3^-.
- In life-threatening acidosis, 1/4 to 1/3 of the deficit can be corrected in the first hour with careful monitoring.
- Aim to correct one-third to one-half of the deficit in approximately 6 to 12 hours and reevaluate clinical signs and acid–base and electrolyte status.
- The bicarbonate deficit can be corrected with oral and intravenous administration of sodium bicarbonate. Note: administration of large volumes of sodium bicarbonate orally or via feeding tube can cause diarrhea.
- Potassium can be added to the initial intravenous fluid therapy (KCl 20–40 mEq/L) not to exceed a rate of 0.5 mEq/kg/h.
- Serial clinical examinations and monitoring for hypernatremia, hyperosmolality, acid–base status, hypokalemia and ionized hypocalcemia are indicated.

Data from Stewart AJ. Secondary renal tubular acidosis in a quarter horse gelding. Vet Clin North Am Equine Pract. 2006;22(1):e47-e61. https://doi.org/10.1016/j.cveq.2005.12.024.

---

macaque.[16–18] In humans, the condition is associated with both acute and chronic renal failure and is characterized by complex mental changes and motor disturbances.[19] Accumulation of uremic toxins due to renal failure is thought to play a role in the development of the condition, although the exact pathogenesis is complex.[19]

The first report of UE in a horse was a 13-year-old grade male presented for a 4-day history of progressive anorexia, listlessness and periodic recumbency, head pressing, and seizure-like activity.[16] The mare was found to be markedly azotemic with a blood urea nitrogen of 166 mg/dL (normal 10–27) and creatinine of 8.2 mg/dL (normal 1.0–2.0). Cerebrospinal fluid analysis was unremarkable. Euthanasia was elected and necropsy revealed severe, subacute, bilateral, chronic, diffuse tubule-interstitial nephritis with superimposed acute tubular necrosis resulting in clinical renal failure. Throughout all regions of the brain was reactive astrogliosis or Alzheimer type II astrogliosis without white matter spongiform change similar to the central nervous system lesions seen in equine hepatic encephalopathy.[16]

A 20-year retrospective study of horses examined for renal disease and neurologic signs not attributed to primary neurologic, hepatic, or other diseases revealed that of the 332 horses with renal disease, 5 met the selection criteria for concurrent neurologic signs.[17] Astrocyte swelling was common to the 4 horses examined at necropsy. Antemortem diagnosis of UE in horses has not been reported but should be considered in horses with neurologic signs and renal failure.[17]

Detection of hyperammonemia in horses with renal disease and neurologic signs that do not have concurrent gastrointestinal disease or liver failure may aid in the identification of horses with suspected UE. Hyperammonemia in the absence of other systemic diseases has been attributed to decreased renal excretion, urinary stasis, and urinary tract infection with urease-producing bacteria in other species.[17,20,21] Treatments aimed at addressing hyperammonemia in horses with renal azotemia could mimic those proposed for cats with this condition and could include reduction in dietary protein, lactulose, probiotics, and antibiotics in addition to the treatment of the underlying renal disease.[20] Awareness of this condition in horses with renal failure may assist in early detection and potential treatment.

Hyponatremic Encephalopathy in Foals with Urinary Tract Disorders

Hyponatremia results from the retention of free water or excess loss of sodium. Causes of severe hyponatremia in foals (serum sodium <122 mEq/L) include diarrhea, uroperitoneum, renal disease, rhabdomyolysis, suspected transient pseudohypoaldosteronism, adrenal insufficiency, excessive water intake, and iatrogenic from excessive administration of water enemas and hypotonic fluids.[22] Severe hyponatremia can result in hyponatremic encephalopathy due to the development of cerebral edema. Occurrence of neurologic deficits appears to be dependent on both the severity and rapidity with which the hyponatremia occurs.[23]

In a retrospective study of hyponatremic (serum sodium $\leq$ 125 mEq/L) foals less than 6 months of age (n = 109) admitted to a hospital the most common diagnoses were enterocolitis/colitis (49/109, 45%), pneumonia (11/109, 10%), clinical sepsis (10/109, 9%), uroperitoneum (9/109, 8%), and renal disease (5/109, 5%).[24] 34% (37/109) had neurologic signs at presentation or developed neurologic signs during hospitalization consisting of obtundation, ataxia, seizures, decreased suckle reflex, hyperreactivity, central blindness, head tilt, opisthotonos, continuous chewing/tongue movement, grimacing, head pressing, circling, and comatose mentation. In the final multivariable model, only serum Na$^+$ and BUN concentrations were significantly associated with neurologic signs. The clinical significance of the contribution of BUN is unclear. The presence of neurologic signs in hyponatremic foals was significantly associated with nonsurvival in this study (20 survivors out of 37 foals with neurologic signs (54%) versus 53 survivors of 72 foals without neurologic signs (74%)).[24]

In a retrospective study of Thoroughbred foals less than 3 months of age presenting to an intensive care unit with severe hyponatremia (serum sodium < 122 mEq/L), 15.9% (11/69) presented with neurologic signs attributed to hyponatremic encephalopathy.[22] The most common primary diagnoses in foals with severe hyponatremia were renal disease (18/69, 26%), enterocolitis (16/69, 23%) and uroperitoneum (15/69, 22%). Of the 18 foals with severe hyponatremia due to renal disease, 9 had previously received nephrotoxic drugs including gentamicin, phenylbutazone, and oxytetracycline. Interestingly, all the foals with hyponatremic encephalopathy (n = 11) had renal disease as the primary diagnosis. Fifty of 69 foals (72.5%) survived to discharge. There was no correlation between admit serum sodium concentration and survival to discharge. In contrast to the study by Dunkel and colleagues[22] there was no significant difference in long-term (approximately 1-year) survival between hyponatremic foals with (7/10, 70%) and without (31/40, 78%) hyponatremic encephalopathy.[24]

Severe hyponatremia in foals is a relatively rare condition, for example, foals presenting with severe hyponatremia represented just 4% of the cases (69/1718) presenting to the ICU during the study period in Collins and colleagues[22] However, several points bear emphasizing. First, renal disease may be associated with the development hyponatremic encephalopathy in foals.[22] This is further underscored in a case series of 4 neonatal foals presenting to an ICU for neurologic signs with severe hyponatremia and azotemia suggestive of acute kidney injury[25] and previous cases reported in the literature with renal disease as a primary or secondary diagnosis.[23,25-27]

Potential mechanisms for the development of hyponatremia in renal disease include decreased glomerular filtration rate and water retention, increased sodium loss with renal tubular damage, and (pseudo)hypoaldosteronism.[22] Foals normally consume low sodium mare's milk in excess of 20% of their body weight daily and produce large volumes of hyposthenuric urine. Kidney injury could result in the retention of large volumes of water and/or increased sodium loss. While the retrospective studies and case series[22-25] do not report results of fractional excretion (FE) of sodium, the frequency with which previous treatment with nephrotoxic medications preceded the development of hyponatremic encephalopathy in one study[22] suggests that renal tubular damage may play a role in the pathophysiology of the condition. Measurement of FE of sodium may be helpful in further elucidation of the mechanism.

It is worth pointing out in one case report, Arroyo and colleagues[27] describe a 10-day-old Quarter horse foal with neurologic signs and severe hyponatremia and hypochloremia. The foal was diagnosed with hydronephrosis/hydroureters, pyelonephritis, and suspected transient pseudohypoaldosteronism. Pseudohypoaldosteronism is thought to occur secondary to pyelonephritis and urinary tract obstruction that causes transient unresponsiveness of the distal tubule to the action of aldosterone. Measurement of serum aldosterone and renin if performed would be expected to be markedly elevated in this condition.[27]

Regardless of how hyponatremic encephalopathy develops in renal disease in foals, prompt recognition and treatment are warranted. Children seem to be more sensitive than adults to the development of hyponatremic encephalopathy owing to their relatively high brain volume-to-cranial vault size ratio resulting in less space to accommodate increases in brain volume that occur with cerebral edema secondary to hyponatremia.[28] Perhaps the same phenomenon exists in horses and explains why foals are more susceptible to hyponatremic encephalopathy than adults, but imaging studies would be required for confirmation.

It is reported that in humans, severe complications of hyponatremia develop when serum sodium decreases at a rate greater than 0.5 mEq/L/h[29] Hypotonic hyponatremia causes the entry of water into the brain resulting in cerebral edema (**Fig. 2**). The surrounding cranium limits expansion of the brain, resulting in intracranial hypertension, and risk of brain injury. Solutes leave the brain tissues within hours inducing water loss and reducing brain swelling.[30] This rapid adaptation explains why neurologic clinical signs are not observed even in cases of severe hyponatremia if it occurs relatively slowly. It is also important to recognize that rapid correction of a sodium deficit in chronic hyponatremia can lead to cellular dehydration and potential to develop osmotic demyelination syndrome.[23]

Osmotic demyelination syndrome is a rare but serious complication of correction of hyponatremia by any method that occurs days to weeks following treatment. Shrinkage of the brain triggers the demyelination of the pontine and extrapontine neurons resulting in mild to severe neurologic dysfunction and in rare cases death.[30] To the author's knowledge, osmotic demyelination syndrome has not been described in horses, but slow correction of chronic hyponatremia in horses is justified.

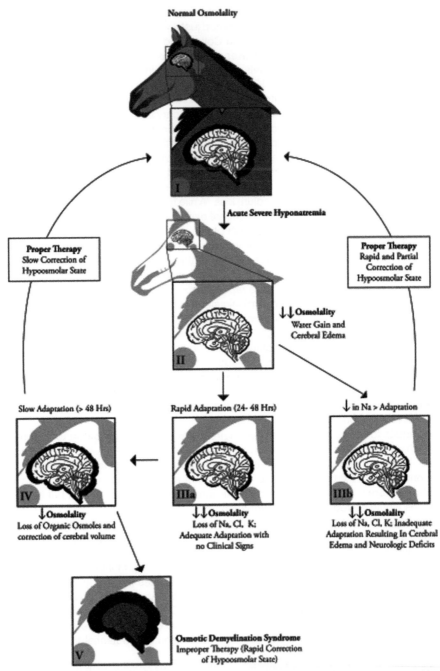

Fig. 2. Effects of hyponatremia on the brain, water balance, and adaptive responses. (I) In healthy states, the body maintains a normal osmolality and tightly regulates cell volume. (II) Shortly after an acute decrease in serum osmolality (ie, hyponatremia), intracellular water accumulates leading to cerebral edema and decreased osmolality in the brain. (IIIa) Rapid adaptation occurs within hours by loss of cellular electrolytes resulting in the reduction of cerebral edema with no neurologic deficits. Alternatively, (IIIb) if the decrease in

While there is no consensus about the optimal treatment of symptomatic hyponatremia in humans, "correction should be of a sufficient pace and magnitude to reverse the manifestations of hypotonicity but not be so rapid and large as to pose a risk of the development of osmotic demyelination."[30]

One treatment protocol in patients with hyponatremic encephalopathy with neurologic signs suggestive of early cerebral edema (nausea, vomiting, and headache) is the administration of an intravenous bolus of 3% saline at 2 mL/kg body weight given over 10 minutes. Bolus administration can be repeated 1 to 2 times if signs persist, but the total change in the serum sodium should not exceed 5 mEq/L in the initial 1 to 2 hours and 15 to 20 mEq/L in the first 48 hours of treatment.[28]

A slightly more conservative approach that has been used successfully in foals with hyponatremic encephalopathy[22] is based on the Adrogué formula.[30] This formula estimates the effects of 1 L IV fluids on the patient's serum sodium concentration (**Box 2**). Foals received 3% hypertonic saline administered via infusion pump and the remainder of their fluid requirements was met with 10% dextrose in water. Ingestion of water and milk was restricted. Once the serum sodium exceeded 120 mEq/L, foals were treated with balanced polyionic crystalloid therapy.[22]

Foals with hyponatremia without encephalopathy were treated similarly to above (n = 6) with 3% hypertonic saline and 10% dextrose in water, but the hyponatremia was corrected more slowly (<0.5 mEq/L/h), or they received isotonic crystalloid fluids (n = 52). All received frequent electrolyte monitoring every 4 to 6 hours.[22]

An alternative approach that has been used successfully in foals with acute hyponatremic encephalopathy is to calculate the amount of sodium required to initially reach a serum concentration of 120 to 125 mEq/L and provide this amount rapidly to prevent further cerebral edema.[25] Then slowly provide the remainder of the deficit required to reach a serum sodium concentration of 132 mEq/L at a rate not to exceed 0.5 mEq/h (see **Box 2**). Careful monitoring of serum sodium levels during treatment is warranted due to difficulty in accounting for ongoing losses and redistribution through the extracellular and intracellular spaces.

Hyponatremic encephalopathy is an uncommon condition that can occur secondary to acute renal failure and other causes in foals. The practitioner should suspect this condition in foals presenting with central neurologic signs. Prompt treatment and careful monitoring are warranted. Prognosis is generally favorable.

Calcium, Phosphorus, and Vitamin D Disorders and Renal Disease

Unique features of calcium, phosphorus, and vitamin D homeostasis in horses are relevant to the discussion of metabolic disorders associated with renal disease.

---

cellular osmolality exceeds the body's adaptive response to rapid loss of electrolytes, cerebral edema persists resulting in acute neurologic deficits. Proper therapy with rapid administration of sodium increases serum osmolality to a subnormal level resulting in decreased cerebral edema and elimination or reduction of neurologic deficits. (IV) Slow (>48 hours) loss of organic osmoles further compensates for a hyposmotic state. Low cellular osmolality persists despite normalization of brain volume. Proper therapy with slow correction of sodium results in a gradual return to normal osmolality. (V) Improper therapy associated with rapid sodium supplementation in chronic hyponatremia results in rapid cell dehydration and the potential to develop osmotic demyelination syndrome. (*From* Wong DM, Sponseller BY, Brokus C et al. Neurologic deficits associated with severe hyponatremia in 2 foals. J Vet Emerg Crit Care 2007;17:275–285; with permission.)

Box 2
Estimation of sodium deficit and initial treatment plan for hyponatremic encephalopathy

Approach for correction of hyponatremia in foals with signs of encephalopathy

Change in serum Na⁺[mEq / L]with 1L of IV fluids

$$= \frac{\left(Na^+ \text{ in IV fluids } \left[mEq/_L\right] \; -- \; measured \; serum \; Na^+[mEq/L] \right)}{(0.6 \; x \; body \; weight \; [kg] + 1)}$$

- Aim to raise the serum sodium concentration by approximately 1.0 to 1.5 mEq/L/h for the first 3h, not to exceed 10 to 12 mEq/L in the first 24h.
- Reassess patient status and serum sodium every 4–6h.
- The remainder of the calculated fluid requirement provided can be by 10% dextrose in water.

Fluid Choice	Sodium Concentration [mEq/L]
7.2% Sodium chloride	1232
5% Sodium chloride	855
0.9% Sodium chloride	154
Plasmalyte A	140
Normasol R	140
Lactated Ringer's solution	130
0.45% Sodium chloride	77
5% Dextrose in water	0

An alternative approach involves the calculation of the amount of sodium required to correct the deficit,

$$Na^+ \text{ required } [mEq] = \left(Na^+ desired \left[mEq/_L\right] \; -- \; measured \; serum \; Na^+ \left[mEq/_L\right] \right.$$
$$\left. \times \right) x \; 0.6 \; x \; body \; weight \; [kg].$$

- Calculate the sodium required to initially reach a serum concentration of 120 to 125 mEq/L.
- In acute hyponatremia, this initial correction should occur rapidly to prevent further cerebral edema.
- Then the sodium required to reach a serum sodium concentration of 132 mmol/L may be provided slowly not to exceed 0.5 mEq/h.
- Reassess patient status and serum sodium every 4-6h.

Data from Collins NM, Axon JE, Carrick JB, Russell CM, Palmer JE. Severe hyponatraemia in foals: clinical findings, primary diagnosis and outcome. Aust Vet J. 2016;94(6):186-191. https://doi.org/10.1111/avj.12446; Hardefeldt LY. Hyponatraemic encephalopathy in azotaemic neonatal foals: four cases. Aust Vet J. 2014;92(12):488-491. https://doi.org/10.1111/avj.12265; Wong DM, Sponseller BY, Brokus C et al. Neurologic deficits associated with severe hyponatremia in 2 foals. J Vet Emerg Crit Care 2007;17:275–285.

Horses lack 1α-hydroxylase in the kidney that converts vitamin D to its most active form, calcitriol.[31] Hence, diseases that affect renal proximal tubular function (ie, Fanconi syndrome) in horses are unlikely to induce hypovitaminosis D. Intestinal absorption of calcium in horses is largely independent of vitamin D. Horses absorb much larger amounts of calcium in their diet compared with other species (up to 75% of dietary calcium).[32] Intestinal absorption of calcium is promoted by acidifying substances and inhibited by compounds that chelate calcium (oxalates, phosphates, and phytates) Renal excretion is the major mechanism for excreting excess dietary calcium in horses.[32]

Hypercalcemia is a common finding in horses with chronic renal failure due to decreased excretion. Hypercalcemia can also occur with neoplasia, hyperparathyroidism, and vitamin D intoxication.[33] Hypercalcemia occurs less commonly in acute renal failure. Causes of hypocalcemia related to renal disease include acute kidney injury, and blister beetle (cantharidin) toxicosis likely due to the loss of calcium via the gastrointestinal tract and kidneys.

Hypervitaminosis D occurs in horses can occur due to the ingestion of calcinogenic plants as well as the administration/ingestion of vitamin D2 and D3.[32,34–36] While hypercalcemia is variable in hypervitaminosis D, hyperphosphatemia is the most consistent laboratory finding.[32] Mineral deposits in the kidneys lead to renal failure. Weight loss, poor appetite, and lameness due to soft tissue mineralization are other findings.[32] Treatment is aimed at reducing calcium and phosphorus intake.[34] Glucocorticoids decrease intestinal absorption, decrease bone resorption and increase urine excretion of calcium, but have limited efficacy in the treatment of hypervitaminosis D.[32]

Findings of nephrocalcinosis along with generalized osteochondrosis and osteoporosis have been associated with chronic zinc and cadmium toxicosis in 2 foals and the dam of one of the foals that resided near a zinc smelter.[37] The foals were examined for lameness, joint swelling, and thriftiness. The foals were euthanized and zinc and cadmium concentrations were markedly elevated in the pancreas, liver, and kidneys. Nephrocalcinosis and osteoporosis consistent with chronic cadmium toxicosis and severe generalized osteochondrosis consistent with chronic zinc toxicosis were observed.[37]

A case series of 5 horses presenting with myopathy, malaise, mild fever, stiffness, hyperfibrinogenemia, hyperphosphatemia, and increased calcium–phosphorus product (Ca*P) had signs consistent with systemic calcinosis and calciphylaxis, conditions not previously described in horses.[38] Although serum vitamin D levels were not determined, there was no known exposure to calcinogenic plants or toxic levels of vitamin D in the horses included in the study and herdmates were not affected. All horses in this case series were euthanized due to the severity of the disease. While mild to moderate azotemia was present in 2/5 horses, the condition described in this case series most closely resembled nonuremic systemic calcinosis.[38]

Calcinosis in humans is characterized by mineralization in the connective tissue of all organs and an elevated serum calcium–phosphorus product (Ca*P). In humans, systemic calcinosis is commonly associated with chronic renal failure but can be due to nonuremic causes.[38] Systemic calcinosis is not commonly observed in horses with chronic renal failure likely because hypophosphatemia (not hyperphosphatemia) is more frequently encountered in horses with chronic renal failure, resulting in a normal serum Ca*P. Calciphylaxis is characterized by small vessel and extravascular calcification and thrombosis.[38]

Idiopathic arterial medial calcification of the thoracic arteries was found in an adult horse with chronic muscle atrophy and stiffness.[39] Differential diagnoses in humans with this condition include hypervitaminosis D, chronic renal disease, diabetes mellitus, hyperparathyroidism, and idiopathic arterial calcification.[39] A cause for this condition could not be identified in this horse.

The pathogenesis of calcinosis, calciphylaxis, and arterial medial calcification in horses remains unclear, and an underlying etiology has not been determined. Treatment would depend on the identification of a particular cause and symptomatic treatment in horses has not been successful.[38,39] It is worth mentioning that glucocorticoid administration may enhance vascular calcification.[40] Glucocorticoids were administered to 3 of 6 horses with reported calcinosis and calciphylaxis. Their role, if any, in disease progression is unknown.[38,39] Practitioners should suspect this condition in horses presenting with malaise, fever, muscle wasting, high serum muscle enzymes, hyperphosphatemia, and elevated Ca*P.

SUMMARY

This article provided an overview of various metabolic disorders associated with renal disease. Examples of diseases associated with acid–base disorders, reduced renal clearance of uremic toxins, reduced excretion of free water or excess sodium loss, and calcium and phosphorus balance highlight the key role the kidneys play in a variety of homeostatic functions.

DISCLOSURE

The author has nothing to disclose.

REFERENCES

1. Palmer BF, Kelepouris E, Clegg DJ. Renal tubular acidosis and management strategies: a narrative review. Adv Ther 2021;38(2):949–68.
2. Kashoor I, Batlle D. Proximal renal tubular acidosis with and without Fanconi syndrome. Kidney Res Clin Pract 2019;38(3):267–81.
3. Aleman MR, Kuesis B, Schott HC, Carlson GP. Renal tubular acidosis in horses (1980-1999). J Vet Intern Med 2001;15(2):136–43.
4. Arroyo LG, Stämpfli HR. Equine renal tubular disorders. Vet Clin North Am Equine Pract 2007;23(3):631, vi.
5. Gull T. Type 1 renal tubular acidosis in a broodmare. Vet Clin North Am Equine Pract 2006;22(1):229–37.
6. MacLeay JM, Wilson JH. Type-II renal tubular acidosis and ventricular tachycardia in a horse. J Am Vet Med Assoc 1998;212(10):1597–9.
7. Ohmes CM, Davis EG, Beard LA, Vander Werf KA, Bianco AW, Giger U. Transient Fanconi syndrome in Quarter horses. Can Vet J 2014;55(2):147–51.
8. O'Leary Hansen T. Renal tubular acidosis in a mare. Compend Contin Educ Pract Vet 1986;8:864–6.
9. Stewart AJ. Secondary renal tubular acidosis in a quarter horse gelding. Vet Clin North Am Equine Pract 2006;22(1):e47–61.
10. Trotter GW, Miller D, Parks A, Arden W. Type II renal tubular acidosis in a mare. J Am Vet Med Assoc 1986;188(9):1050–1.
11. van der Kolk JH, Kalsbeek HC. Renal tubular acidosis in a mare. Vet Rec 1993; 133(2):43–4.
12. van der Kolk JH. Renale tubulaire acidose (type 2) bij een friese merrie [Renal tubular acidosis (type 2) in a Friesian mare]. Tijdschr Diergeneeskd 1994; 119(22):675–6.
13. van der Kolk JH, de Graaf-Roelfsema E, Joles JA, et al. Mixed proximal and distal renal tubular acidosis without aminoaciduria in a mare. J Vet Intern Med 2007; 21(5):1121–5.
14. Ziemer EL, Parker HR, Carlson GP, Smith BP, Ishizaki G. Renal tubular acidosis in two horses: diagnostic studies. J Am Vet Med Assoc 1987;190(3):289–93.

15. Ziemer EL, Parker HR, Carlson GP, Smith BP. Clinical features and treatment of renal tubular acidosis in two horses. J Am Vet Med Assoc 1987;190(3):294–6.

16. Bouchard PR, Weldon AD, Lewis RM, Summers BA. Uremic encephalopathy in a horse. Vet Pathol 1994;31(1):111–5.

17. Frye MA, Johnson JS, Traub-Dargatz JL, Savage CJ, Fettman MJ, Gould DH. Putative uremic encephalopathy in horses: five cases (1978-1998). J Am Vet Med Assoc 2001;218(4):560–6.

18. Mustonen A, Gonzalez O, Mendoza E, Kumar S, Dick EJ Jr. Uremic encephalopathy in a rhesus macaque (Macaca mulatta): a case report and a brief review of the veterinary literature [published online ahead of print, 2018 Apr 25]. J Med Primatol 2018. https://doi.org/10.1111/jmp.12348.

19. Seifter JL, Samuels MA. Uremic encephalopathy and other brain disorders associated with renal failure. Semin Neurol 2011;31(2):139–43.

20. Carvalho L, Kelley D, Labato MA, Webster CR. Hyperammonemia in azotemic cats [published online ahead of print, 2020 Nov 20]. J Feline Med Surg 2020. https://doi.org/10.1177/1098612X20972039. 1098612X20972039.

21. Hall JA, Allen TA, Fettman MJ. Hyperammonemia associated with urethral obstruction in a dog. J Am Vet Med Assoc 1987;191(9):1116–8.

22. Collins NM, Axon JE, Carrick JB, Russell CM, Palmer JE. Severe hyponatraemia in foals: clinical findings, primary diagnosis and outcome. Aust Vet J 2016;94(6):186–91.

23. Wong DM, Sponseller BY, Brokus C, et al. Neurologic deficits associated with severe hyponatremia in 2 foals. J Vet Emerg Crit Care 2007;17:275–85.

24. Dunkel B, Dodson F, Chang YM, Slovis NM. Retrospective evaluation of the association between hyponatremia and neurological dysfunction in hospitalized foals (2012-2016): 109 cases. J Vet Emerg Crit Care (San Antonio) 2020;30(1):66–73.

25. Hardefeldt LY. Hyponatraemic encephalopathy in azotaemic neonatal foals: four cases. Aust Vet J 2014;92(12):488–91.

26. Zicker SC, Marty GD, Carlson GP, et al. Bilateral renal dysplasia with nephron hypoplasia in a foal. J Am Vet Med Assoc 1990;196:2001–5.

27. Arroyo LG, Vengust M, Dobson H, Viel L. Suspected transient pseudohypoaldosteronism in a 10-day-old quarter horse foal. Can Vet J 2008;49(5):494–8.

28. Achinger SG, Ayus JC. Treatment of Hyponatremic Encephalopathy in the Critically Ill. Crit Care Med 2017;45(10):1762–71.

29. Cluitmans FH, Meinders AE. Management of severe hyponatremia: rapid or slow correction? Am J Med 1990;88(2):161–6.

30. Adrogué HJ, Madias NE. Hyponatremia. N Engl J Med 2000;342(21):1581–9.

31. Breidenbach A, Schlumbohm C, Harmeyer J. Peculiarities of vitamin D and of the calcium and phosphate homeostatic system in horses. Vet Res 1998;29(2):173–86.

32. Toribio RE. Disorders of calcium and phosphate metabolism in horses. Vet Clin North Am Equine Pract 2011;27(1):129–47.

33. Toribio RE, Kohn CW, Rourke KM, Levine AL, Rosol TJ. Effects of hypercalcemia on serum concentrations of magnesium, potassium, and phosphate and urinary excretion of electrolytes in horses. Am J Vet Res 2007;68(5):543–54.

34. Harmeyer J, Schlumbohm C. Effects of pharmacological doses of Vitamin D3 on mineral balance and profiles of plasma Vitamin D3 metabolites in horses. J Steroid Biochem Mol Biol 2004;89-90(1–5):595–600.

35. Harrington DD, Page EH. Acute vitamin D3 toxicosis in horses: case reports and experimental studies of the comparative toxicity of vitamins D2 and D3. J Am Vet Med Assoc 1983;182(12):1358–69.

36. Harrington DD. Acute vitamin D2 (ergocalciferol) toxicosis in horses: case report and experimental studies. J Am Vet Med Assoc 1982;180(8):867–73.
37. Gunson DE, Kowalczyk DF, Shoop CR, Ramberg CF Jr. Environmental zinc and cadmium pollution associated with generalized osteochondrosis, osteoporosis, and nephrocalcinosis in horses. J Am Vet Med Assoc 1982;180(3):295–9.
38. Tan JY, Valberg SJ, Sebastian MM, et al. Suspected systemic calcinosis and calciphylaxis in 5 horses. Can Vet J 2010;51(9):993–9.
39. Fales-Williams A, Sponseller B, Flaherty H. Idiopathic arterial medial calcification of the thoracic arteries in an adult horse. J Vet Diagn Invest 2008;20(5):692–7.
40. Kirton JP, Wilkinson FL, Canfield AE, Alexander MY. Dexamethasone downregulates calcification-inhibitor molecules and accelerates osteogenic differentiation of vascular pericytes: implications for vascular calcification. Circ Res 2006; 98(10):1264–72.

Imaging of the Urinary Tract

Marta Cercone, DVM, PhD

KEYWORDS

- Horse • Urinary tract • Endoscopy • Ultrasonography • Computed tomography
- Scintigraphy

KEY POINTS

- Equine urinary tract imaging should always complement physical examination and laboratory tests in case of hematuria, stranguria, and incontinence.
- Urinary endoscopy is crucial when investigating hematuria and hemospermia.
- Ultrasonography allows to evaluate the renal parenchyma and vascularization, guiding in obtaining targeted biopsy.
- A diagnosis of distal urolithiasis should always be accompanied by evaluation of the entire urinary tract to rule out nephrolithiasis and pyelonephritis.
- Computed tomographic urography is the ideal diagnostic in foals with suspected urinary congenital abnormalities.
- Valuable information on renal function is obtained through Doppler ultrasonography and nuclear scintigraphy.

▶ Video content accompanies this article at http://www.vetequine.theclinics.com

INTRODUCTION

Imaging is fundamental in discriminating between pathologies of the equine urinary system, guiding treatment and prognostic assessment. Ultrasonography has become the screening modality of choice because of its noninvasiveness and accessibility. Endoscopy is elected when evaluating hematuria, whereas Doppler ultrasonography and nuclear scintigraphy can help assess renal function. Contrast studies are conducted radiographically or with computed tomography (CT) to determine urinary tract integrity or congenital malformation in foals and miniature horses. Laparoscopy is described elsewhere in this issue, with retroperitoneoscopy for direct visualization of the equine kidneys.[1]

ENDOSCOPY

Endoscopy of the equine urinary tract requires a flexible endoscope (<12 mm diameter in adults, >1 m length), and smaller diameters are optimal for foals and ureteral

Department of Clinical Sciences, Cornell University, 930 Campus Road, Ithaca, NY 14853, USA
E-mail address: mc957@cornell.edu

Vet Clin Equine 38 (2022) 123–140
https://doi.org/10.1016/j.cveq.2021.11.009
0749-0739/22/© 2021 Elsevier Inc. All rights reserved.

vetequine.theclinics.com

endoscopy. Sedation helps relax the penis in adult horses, but the risk of permanent penile dysfunction when using acepromazine and the increase in urine production following α_2-agonists, transiently altering urine characteristics, should be taken into account. The endoscope should be sterilized, and penis/vulva thoroughly cleaned with dilute chlorhexidine or povidone-iodine. Passage through the urethra is facilitated using sterile nonspermicidal lubricant gel and intermittent air inflation; advancement should be gentle and slow to identify focal abnormalities. Endoscopy is crucial in identifying the source of hematuria,[2,3] but sometimes defects are not diagnosed because of small size or equipment limitations.[4] Normal urethral mucosa is pale pink with longitudinal folds, and submucosal vasculature is prominent toward the bladder.[5] Urethral mucosa can become hyperemic as air is inflated, so it must be evaluated as the scope advances. Urinary catheterization before endoscopy can induce erythematous mucosa and air bubbles, to be differentiated from preexisting lesions. In males, the pelvic urethra widens into the ampulla, where bulbourethral glands openings are visualized dorsally in two parallel rows (**Fig. 1**), and cranially, the colliculus seminalis where the ejaculatory and prostatic ducts open. Rents, tears, and varicosity of the proximal urethra, most common on the dorsocaudal aspect in the pelvic and ischial portion, cause hematuria in geldings and hemospermia in stallions (Video 1).[6,7] Linear defects are often identified without evidence of inflammation or hemorrhage.[5] Chronic hematuria may occur with fistulated lesions communicating with the corpus spongiosum. Strictures secondary to trauma, surgery, or calculus obstruction appear as urethral narrowing that cannot be distended with air.[8] Small cystic calculi can lodge in the urethra as it narrows over the ischial arch, causing inflammation and ulceration (**Fig. 2**). Incomplete obstruction results in dysuria, whereas complete obstruction can lead to bladder rupture unless diagnosed and corrected promptly.[9,10] The entire urinary tract should be evaluated in horses diagnosed with distal urolithiasis, because many have calculi in multiple locations and the condition is secondary to pyelonephritis with impaired renal function.[11,12] Urethral narrowing or obstruction can also result from neoplasia originating from the urethra itself or external genitalia.

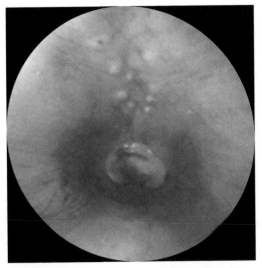

Fig. 1. Endoscopic image of the pelvic urethra, ampullar portion. The openings of the bulbourethral glands are visualized dorsally in two parallel rows, and more cranially in the center of the image is the colliculus seminalis.

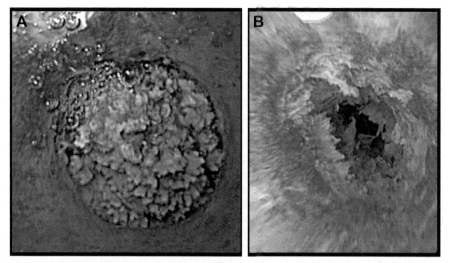

Fig. 2. Endoscopic image of a urethral calculus in a 14-year-old quarter horse gelding. (*A*) A spiculated calculus (calcium carbonate) causes complete obstruction of the urethra at the level of the ischial arch. (*B*) Pressure necrosis and peripheral inflamed mucosa are detected on the obstruction site after removal of the calculus via perineal urethrostomy.

Once the endoscope is passed through the urethral sphincter, the bladder is distended with air to examine its internal surface. Discomfort and iatrogenic bladder rupture have been reported with large volumes of air.[13] Rare cystoscopy-related air embolisms have been described in humans and horses,[14–17] involving the passage of air through the mucosa into the venous circulation, which is directly related to air volume, rate of accumulation,[18] and the position of the bladder relative to the heart. Typical clinical signs include sudden agitation, dysrhythmia, cardiovascular collapse, and neurologic signs (ataxia, blindness, and seizures). Air trapped within the right ventricle and pulmonary vasculature induces myocardial ischemia, hyperacute inflammation with pulmonary edema, and cerebral hypoxia. Diagnosis is presumptive but could be confirmed via ultrasonographic visualization of air bubbles within the right heart and vasculature. In cases of severe cystitis, with a compromised mucosal barrier, insufflation of carbon dioxide (absorbed and excreted more rapidly), preoxygenation, and anticoagulants are used preventatively.[16]

The normal bladder has a smooth, glistening, pale pink mucosa, with visible submucosal vasculature. Cystoscopy enables assessment of mucosal thickness, damage (erosion, ulcers, necrosis), masses, cystoliths, and sabulous accumulation.[19–23] Hemorrhage, ecchymosis, and sludge material are found with cystitis.[24] Cystoliths cause bladder erythema and inflammation, with mucosal erosions and consequent dysuria and hematuria, particularly after exercise.[25–29] Cystoscopy is fundamental during initial diagnostics; after surgical urolith removal; when searching for fragments or bladder tears; and, considering the high recurrence rate, as long-term follow-up.[10,26] Although more common in foals, bladder rupture can also occur in mares following parturition. Endoscopy can identify the number and location of tears and guide surgical repair.[27] Sabulous urolithiasis describes accumulation of sediment (primarily calcium carbonate crystals) in the ventral aspect of the bladder; it may be a consequence, not a cause, of urinary incontinence.[20,22,28] Although cystoliths are typically found in poorly filled bladders, sabulous urolithiasis occurs with large, atonic bladders, suggestive of bladder dysfunction. The persistent sediment causes mucosal damage and cystitis, with irregular, raised areas intermixed with depressed hemorrhagic, ulcerative spots, and secondary infection.[29] Ulcerative cystitis is rarely a primary condition in horses, usually secondary to calculi, phenylbutazone administration, cantharidin toxicity, or urinary obstruction from causes external to the urinary tract.[5,30,31] Idiopathic hemorrhagic cystitis is characterized by hemorrhagic and thickened mucosa with proliferative lesions over the cranioventral or apical region that can extend peripherally.[32] Proliferative and multinodular bladder lesions could also be neoplastic, with squamous cell carcinoma being the most frequently reported,[33] followed by transitional cell carcinomas, lymphosarcomas, leiomyosarcomas, and fibromatous polyps.[34–36] A transendoscopic biopsy is needed to differentiate between these causes of hematuria and stranguria.

Cystoscopy should be included in the assessment of incontinence to diagnose and guide surgical treatment of ectopic ureters in young horses.[37] The ureteral openings appear as slitlike clefts dorsal to the trigone (at 10 and 2 o'clock) through which urine passes approximately once every minute. A polyethylene tube can be passed through the endoscope instrument channel for individual ureter catheterization and urine sampling, and advanced to the renal pelvis under ultrasonography guidance.[5,38,39] If the ureteral openings cannot be visualized within the bladder, dyes that discolor urine (sodium fluorescein or azosulfamide) administered intravenously help locate the ectopic ureteral opening within the pelvic urethra (or vagina and uterus in females).[40–43] Ureteral ectopia rarely occurs in horses, but when present, urinary incontinence with urine scalding is seen from birth.[37,41–43] Endoscopy visualizes the distal opening of the ectopic ureter, requiring a contrast study and ultrasonography to evaluate possible renal agenesis, hydronephrosis, and hydroureter.[44] Visualization of the ureter opening without urine flow indicates obstruction, as in ureterolithiasis, when the opening can also appear edematous, inflamed, irregular, and fibrotic, or dilated with mucous or blood plugs (**Fig. 3**).[11,45] At the site of obstruction, the ureteral mucosa shows erosion,

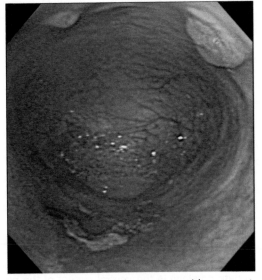

Fig. 3. Cystoscopy of a 15-year-old quarter horse mare with recurrent urolithiasis. A small amount of sediment is pooling ventrally, associated with focal mucosal inflammation. The openings of the ureters are visualized dorsally; note the edematous, enlarged, and misshapen opening of the right ureter.

ulcers, and necrosis (Video 2), whereas passage of thick discolored urine suggests pyelonephritis, often secondary to urolithiasis, recurrent cystitis, and bladder paralysis.[12,46] Chronic bacterial infection and papillary necrosis may provide foci for
nephrolith formation, but establishing whether urolithiasis or infection developed first
is often impossible.[47] Hemorrhagic discharge from the ureter can result from nephrolithiasis, pyelonephritis, renal neoplasia, or idiopathic renal hemorrhage.[3]

Long, small-diameter endoscopes allow ureteropyeloscopy (Video 2).[48] A flexible
guidewire or polyethylene tube is passed into the ureteral opening, advanced approximately 10 cm, followed by the endoscope. Passage is easy in pathologically distended ureters; otherwise, saline infusion can dilate the lumen. The ureter has pale
yellow epithelium, with longitudinal folds and peristalsis. Approaching the renal pelvis,
the renal crest and terminal recesses are observed, with regular contraction of the
pelvis initiating the propulsion of urine along the ureter.[48]

Endoscopy allows targeted biopsy of intraluminal focal lesions, and chromoendoscopy, by spraying dyes over the mucosa, highlights mucosal anomalies optimizing
collection of significative biopsies.[19,49] The stains used, such as methylene blue, are
absorbed into tissue and pretreating the mucosa with a mucolytic (N-acetylcysteine
or acetic acid) results in higher contrast of the epithelium.[49] Recently, chromoendoscopy of normal bladder and cystitis have been described in female donkeys and
correlated to histopathologic findings.[19]

ULTRASONOGRAPHY

Ultrasonography is the method of choice for imaging renal parenchyma to evaluate
hematuria of renal origin, nephrolithiasis, renal failure, and pyelonephritis.[3,50] Transcutaneous ultrasound can visualize the kidneys through a transabdominal[51–53] or translumbar[54] approach, whereas the bladder, distal ureters, and urethra are evaluated
transrectally. A 2- to 5-MHz transducer (convex or phased array) provides the best
penetration with adequate resolution; however, frequency, gain, and depth settings
depend on the individual machine and patient.[55] Poor ultrasonographic definition is
common in obese, gray, or draft horses. The left kidney (typical bean shape) is visualized between the left fifteenth intercostal space and paralumbar fossa, whereas the
right kidney (triangular or horseshoe shape) is found consistently in the fifteenth to
seventeenth right intercostal space. Because the left kidney is medial to the spleen,
obtaining high-quality transabdominal images is often difficult, thereby a translumbar
approach has been described to visualize both kidneys from the lateral margin of the
transverse processes.[54] Reference size measures in Thoroughbred horses are comparable between techniques and correlate with anatomic ex vivo measurements;
the average length of both kidneys ranges 15 to 18 cm, whereas the right kidney is
larger in width (13.4–14 cm) and depth (6.7–7.4 cm).[52,54,56]

Ultrasound can image the renal capsule, cortex, medulla, renal pelvis, intrarenal
vessels, collecting system, and proximal ureter. Different echogenicity and echotexture characterize each area, and pathologic changes are detected by comparing those
characteristics with the spleen and liver, subjectively or quantitatively.[57] The capsule,
a smooth hyperechoic line, encloses the renal cortex (~ 1–1.4 cm thick, with a fine
texture homogeneously echogenic), whereas the medulla is hypoechoic to
anechoic.[52,54] The renal pelvis, with fat and connective tissue, appears as a hyperechoic central band. Interlobar or arcuate vessels are small, regular anechoic areas
with echogenic rims, identifiable with color Doppler, which helps detecting and char-
acterizing regional hemodynamics. Color flow Doppler ultrasonography helps diagnosing vascular anomalies predisposing hematuria, whereas absence of blood flow

in cortical lesions suggests infarction.[58,59] Intrarenal arterial flow interrelates with renal function, and altered renal perfusion represents an early sign of impaired kidney function in humans and small animals.[60] Pulsed wave Doppler ultrasound is used to quantify renal perfusion by calculating the renal resistivity index (RRI) and pulsatility index. The systolic peak velocity and end diastolic velocity of the arcuate arteries in normal horses and foals has been studied, and the resulting RRI ranged from 0.48 to 0.58.[61,62] RRI greater than 0.7 is indicative of renal pathology in other species[60]; indeed, it increases in acute tubular necrosis, acute interstitial diseases, and renal obstruction.[61] RRI seems more sensitive in identifying nephropathy than traditional B-mode ultrasound and could be useful to assess the progression of renal injury and establish a prognosis.[60] Unfortunately, current RRI data in horses diagnosed with acute kidney injury seem inconsistent.[63]

On the kidney medial aspect, the hilum is identified by the renal artery and vein, and the peristaltic ureter with its hypoechoic wall. Depending on the horse size, the adrenal glands are visualized craniomedial to the kidneys. Ultrasound is essential in guiding biopsies of kidneys or perirenal masses,[64–66] allowing accurate identification of the target abnormalities. In diffuse and bilateral diseases, the preferred biopsy site is the lateral portion of the right kidney, guided by transverse imaging through the seventeenth intercostal space. Ultrasound-guided biopsy is safe, with reported transient hematuria but rarely clinically significant pain or hemorrhage.[65,67]

The bladder is visualized in the ventrocaudal abdomen, with an echoic, smooth wall, approximately 5 mm thick depending on distention.[55,68] Urine appears echoic from calcium carbonate crystals; when sedimented, resuspension of the crystals by gentle balloting with the transducer helps rule out a pathologic sabulous urolithiasis. Transcutaneous ultrasonography in males should include the urethra along its perineal and penile length, using a high-frequency (6–10 MHz) linear or microconvex transducer. The urethra is enclosed by the urethralis muscle and the bulbourethral glands over the ischial arch, and distally by the bulbospongiosus muscle with the corpus spongiosum. The urethra has approximately 1.0- to 1.5-cm diameter in the perineal and penile portion, with a usually obliterated lumen when inactive.

Anatomic references for transcutaneous ultrasonography of the urinary system in foals and adults are similar, but in neonates, a complete ultrasonographic exam should include the urachus and umbilical structures. The foals' smaller size and reduced adipose tissue allow the use of higher frequency transducers (6–10 MHz). Normal size (8–10.5 cm length, 6.7–10.4 cm width) and ultrasonographic characteristics of the kidneys in Thoroughbred neonatal foals have been reported.[69] Medial and cranial to the hilus, the adrenal glands are found between the kidney and caudal vena cava (right) and ventral to the aorta (left).[69,70] In neonatal foals, the renal pelvis and proximal ureters seem dilated, possibly related to their exclusive liquid diet and large volume of urine produced.[69] The bladder is easily evaluated against the ventral abdominal wall. In the neonate, umbilical arteries run along the lateral aspect of the bladder in a cranioaxial and ventral direction, converging to the urachus in an oblong grouping, normally measuring less than 2.5 cm in width, with each umbilical artery less than 1-cm diameter.[71] The urachus, mostly a potential space, should involute after birth when the foal starts voiding urine through the urethra.

Transrectal ultrasonography in the adult horse allows imaging of the left kidney, renal vein and artery and adrenal gland, distal ureters, entire bladder, and pelvic urethra.[55,72] The procedure is well tolerated with or without sedation, with adequate lubrication. Lidocaine 2% intrarectal infusion and intravenous butylscopolamine reduce peristalsis and rectal pressure. The potential muscle-relaxing effect of sedatives and butylscopolamine should be considered if assessing ureteral function.[73] A 6- to 10-

MHz microconvex is the ideal transducer to visualize all relevant organs, whereas a 5-MHz rectal transducer allows evaluation of the distal ureters, urethra, and partially of the left kidney and bladder.[55] The bladder has a round to oval shape depending on urine distention; the trigone and the ureterovesicular junctions are imaged caudally. Transversely, the ureters are circular structures, with hypoechoic walls (1.3–2.4 mm thick) protruding into the dorsal aspect of the bladder; regular pulsatile urine flow is highlighted and evaluated with color Doppler.[74] Transrectal imaging provides the best ureteral visualization but is limited in small or very young horses.[75] In males, the deferent ducts appear as small structures along the bladder wall, like the ureters but lacking peristaltic activity, with a fusiform enlargement in stallions, the ampulla (~2 cm diameter and 15–20 cm length). Further lateral to the ureteral opening the seminal vesicles appear as piriform sacs filled with hypoechoic fluid. The prostate, two lobes (1.7–5.9 cm thick) connected by an isthmus, are visualized over the bladder neck and urethra. Moving caudally, the pelvic urethra (1.5–2.6 cm wide) is surrounded by the urethralis muscle. Males' urethra has an elliptical dilation (~3–5 cm) before narrowing near the ischial arch, where the ovoid bulbourethral glands appear dorsally on either side. The echogenicity of the accessory genital glands varies widely between individuals based on recent sexual activity.

Sonographic Abnormalities

Kidney abnormalities can be capsular or pericapsular, and they can involve the parenchyma (focal, multifocal, or diffuse alterations), the collecting system, and the vasculature. Renal size varies with acute (enlargement) or chronic (contraction with altered shape) renal failure. Perirenal hemorrhage is usually associated with trauma, biopsy, or (rarely) renal rupture,[76] whereas accumulation of hypoechoic to anechoic fluid supports acute renal failure.[56] Many horses in acute renal failure may not show ultrasonographic abnormalities, whereas others have renal enlargement, widening of the cortex, and decreased cortical and medullary echogenicity caused by edema, hyperemia, and interstitial inflammation.[77] Interstitial nephritis, bacterial pyelonephritis, and chronic renal disease present with diffuse increase in echogenicity of cortex and medulla, loss of corticomedullary distinction, heterogeneous areas with focal hyperechogenicity, and abnormal renal outline with lobulation (Video 3).[50,58,78,79] The medullary rim sign is a distinct hyperechoic band parallel to the corticomedullary junction resulting from dystrophic microscopic calcification of the outer zone of the medulla.[53,80] Medullary rim sign is specifically associated with medullary necrosis consequent to decreased renal perfusion from chronic or overdosed nonsteroidal anti-inflammatory drug administration.[81] Increased size and echogenicity of the medulla are attributed to blood in idiopathic renal hematuria.[2] Renal cysts are anechoic structures with thin smooth walls and acoustic enhancement, whereas abscesses and hematomas have irregular margins and echotexture with loculation or septa.[51] More complex lesions with variable echogenicity, mineralization, and shadowing are usually associated with neoplasia.[35,64] Granulomatous lesions are rare findings associated with *Halicephalobus gingivalis* and *Dioctophyme renale* infection, whereas infarction or subcapsular or pelvic hemorrhage is caused by *Strongylus vulgaris* larval migration. Pyelectasia is found in pyelonephritis (echogenic to hyperechoic fluid with floating debris),[59] or in ureteral obstruction or ectopy induced hydronephrosis.[82] In the latter, pelvis and ureter are distended by anechoic fluid, and in severe cases, the calyces are also dilated with compression and thinning of the surrounding parenchyma (**Fig. 4**). In severe chronic pyelonephritis, the kidney can completely lose structure appearing as an abscess (**Fig. 5**).[12] The pelvic recesses are the primary location for nephroliths, which should be ruled out whenever calculi are found in the distal urinary tract.[78,83]

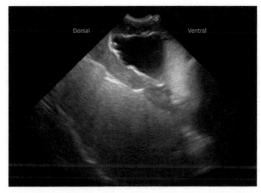

Fig. 4. Transrectal ultrasonographic image of the left kidney in a 14-year-old warmblood gelding diagnosed with bilateral ureterolithiasis. Hydronephrosis with echoic sediment and abnormally thin renal parenchyma, lacking corticomedullary distinction. (*Courtesy* of Dr Meg Turpin.)

Calculi are bright echogenic foci of variable size and shape with acoustic shadow **(Fig. 6)**.[45,84] The sites most prone to calculi obstruction are the ureterovesicular junctions and the ischial urethra; ultrasonographic findings include proximal ectasia, thickened edematous wall, and irregular mucosal surface with possible blood clots **(Fig. 7)**.[43,75] Congenital malformations inducing pollakiuria, dysuria, stranguria, and incontinence are renal hypoplasia, dysplasia, polycystic kidneys, and ectopic ureters.[85–88] Abnormal nephrogenesis causes renal dysplasia, where kidneys appear small and misshapen with poor corticomedullary distinction. Kidneys may produce urine without functioning normally, and are defined as hypoplastic when lacking medullary tissue, or greater than one-third of total parenchyma is lost.[40,66]

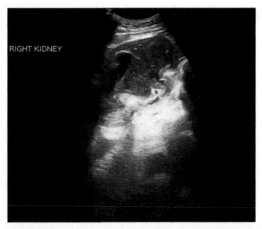

Fig. 5. Ultrasonographic image of the right kidney of a 15-year-old quarter horse mare with pyelonephritis associated with recurrent urolithiasis (see Video 2). Severe renal remodeling resembling an abscess. Note the pyelectasia with amorphous heterogeneous material layered ventrally to anechoic fluid. The surrounding parenchyma is thin with heterogenous echogenicity, and multiple hyperechoic foci.

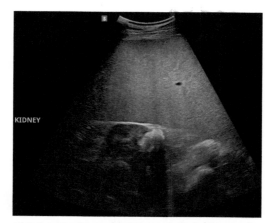

Fig. 6. Ultrasonographic image of a nephrolith in the left kidney of a 15-year-old quarter horse gelding. The horse, presenting with pollakiuria, stranguria, and hematuria, was diagnosed with a cystolith and multiple nephroliths in both kidneys. The left kidney was found to be small (8 × 7 cm), heteroechoic, and lacking corticomedullary demarcation.

Rectal palpation and transrectal ultrasonography of the bladder should be performed when investigating stranguria with hematuria to differentiate between cystitis, bladder neoplasia, and cystic calculi.[33] A diverticulum of the bladder or urachus should be ruled out in stranguric foals with distended bladder. A mass effect associated with the bladder wall is consistent with neoplasia or trauma (**Fig. 8**),[21,32,33,36,89–91] whereas diffusely thickened, edematous, and irregular wall, with or without sedimentation, is associated with cystitis.[56] A markedly distended bladder with hyperechoic sediment suggests sabulous urolithiasis,[22] where the sediment can compact into large inspissated spheres.[28] Echoic, highly cellular swirling urine is visualized in hemorrhagic cystitis.[32] Heterogeneous hematomas attached to the wall or floating amorphous echoic clots with smooth edges are found after intracystic hemorrhage.[92,93] Wall defects, surrounded by swollen mucosa, are detected with ruptured bladder, associated with increased hypoechoic peritoneal fluid.[23,26,27] In neonates, tears can involve the

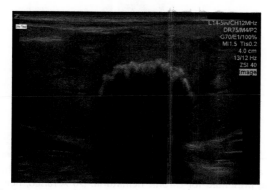

Fig. 7. Transrectal ultrasonographic image of a cystolith in an 11-year-old thoroughbred gelding referred for stranguria. A calculus was found over the pelvic floor, within the bladder neck; note the calculus spiculated surface and the thickened and edematous bladder wall surrounding the stone.

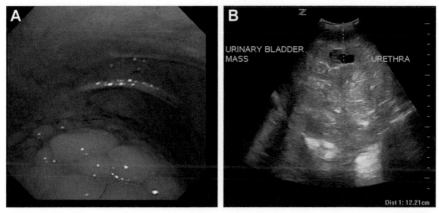

Fig. 8. Endoscopic and transrectal ultrasonographic images of a transitional cell carcinoma in a 21-year-old quarter horse gelding. (*A*) A large multilobulated structure invaded most of the caudal bladder. (*B*) Transrectal ultrasonography confirmed the mass size (12 cm diameter) and its caudal extension surrounding the urethra. (*Courtesy* of Drs Sally DeNotta and Thomas Divers.)

bladder or exclusively the urachus; abdominal wall edema is likely with tear within the umbilical stump.[71,94] Intrabdominal or retroperitoneal accumulation of anechoic urine can develop from ureteral tears, depending on their location.[95,96] In case of bladder rupture without an evident traumatic cause, the urethra should be assessed for obstruction, stricture, compression, or neoplastic infiltration (**Fig. 9**).[31,97] Ultrasonography allows visualization of urethral strictures and real-time monitoring during balloon dilation procedure.[8] Complete ultrasonography of thorax and abdomen should

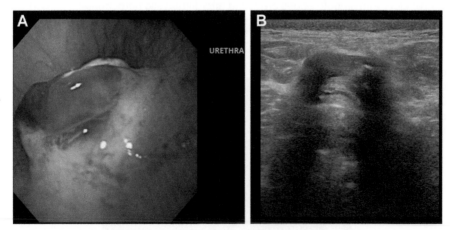

Fig. 9. Endoscopic and transrectal ultrasonographic images of the urethra in a 12-year-old warmblood gelding presented for chronic hematuria. (*A*) A raised, hemorrhagic, nodular mass partially obstructing the lumen of the pelvic urethra. (*B*) Transrectal ultrasonography confirmed the location of the mass exclusively within the urethral wall, showing a heterogenous structure with several well-defined vessels. Transendoscopic biopsy revealed urothelial hyperplasia with Brunn nests and venous telangiectasia.

accompany diagnosis of urinary tract neoplasia to rule out metastasis or extraurinary involvement.

RADIOGRAPHY

Radiography is used rarely to evaluate urinary tract disease in horses.[40] Survey radiographs of the kidney provide little information besides rough size, shape, and position, and intestinal gas makes interpretation even more challenging.[98] Contrast radiographic studies can highlight the ureters, bladder, and urethra mostly in foals. Intravenous urography potentially shows hypoplasia, strictures, or dilatation of collecting system and ureters, providing a global idea about renal function.[82,98] Distal ureter detail is often limited, and the large volume of contrast required can result in nondiagnostic studies.[44] Direct pyelography eludes this limitation by injecting the contrast into the renal pelvis under ultrasonographic guidance.[99] Retrograde contrast studies help evaluate the bladder and ureters when an ectopic ureter is suspected,[41,99] and negative cystogram (pneumocystogram) delineates the shape of the bladder and accentuates the ureteral openings after intravenous urography.[82,100] Despite the potential of contrast radiography, tissue overlap still precludes a complete characterization of anatomic malformation.[100]

COMPUTED TOMOGRAPHY

CT is the gold standard to diagnose urinary stones in humans, whereas multiphasic CT urography allows simultaneous evaluation of vasculature and parenchyma to assess congenital anomalies, trauma, infection, and tumors.[92,98] Although congenital disorders are rare in foals, many cases of ectopic ureter and other anomalies are reported.[37,41–44,75,82,85–87,101] Ectopic ureter diagnosis through other modalities may not completely represent the condition.[102] CT provides the most accurate imaging and exact path of ureters and additional congenital disorders, guiding eventual surgical correction.[37,101] The size of common CT gantry limits imaging in the horse, and traditionally, abdominal CT is impractical in equine patients greater than 136 kg, but urinary CT has been successful also in large foals.[101] Multislice CT urography, compared with intravenous urography, retrograde ureterography, and direct pyelography, is not invasive and can accurately determine ectopic ureters or ureteral tears.[96] Combining endoscopy, ultrasound, and CT is often necessary to evaluate complicated cases with involvement of multiple urinary or extraurinary structures.[75,87,92] Contrast CT has been also used to calculate glomerular filtration rate in a foal.[103] CT features and image acquisition recently described in dogs could be used in foals, such as three-dimensional volume rendering with virtual endoscopy visualization tools, and four-dimensional CT excretory urography.[104,105]

In human medicine MRI is considered complementary to CT providing greater contrast resolution without the risks associated with iodinated contrast or exposure to radiation; quantitative imaging biomarkers are derived to assess fibrosis, inflammation, edema, perfusion, filtration, and tissue oxygenation.[106,107] Besides an ex vivo anatomic evaluation of equine kidneys,[48] no studies evaluated MRI performance in diagnosing urinary disease in foals.

NUCLEAR SCINTIGRAPHY

Scintigraphy displays physiologic processes by evaluating the amount of radioactive agent within a region at a given point in time or over time (dynamic imaging). Scintigraphy is a safe, noninvasive, easy procedure to diagnose urinary anomalies, assess renal function, and determine prognosis. Quantitative renal nuclear medicine estimates glomerular filtration rate and effective renal blood flow, using imaging and non-imaging techniques.[108,109] Functional renal scintigraphy has been validated in horses against such traditional methods as inulin and para-aminohippurate clearance.[51,110] Several radiopharmaceuticals are used in equine scintigraphy that also bind to tubular epithelial cells, providing morphologic details and information on the relative function of the two kidneys. The glomerular filtration rate measured using a gamma camera is less accurate in horses than other species because of depth-related attenuation, difficulties in background correction, and movement.[110] Scintigraphy, providing information on renal vascular perfusion, excretion patterns, and individual kidney function, can detect early renal dysfunction, monitor response to therapy, and provide prognostic information.[110] Despite the extensive literature validating scintigraphic evaluation of renal function in horses, only a few case reports highlight its use in clinical setting.[12,44]

SUMMARY

Imaging techniques should be used coupled with history, clinical examination, and laboratory assessment to fully evaluate horses with suspected urinary tract disease. Endoscopy and ultrasonography are complementary, providing structural and intraluminal information and, facilitating biopsy, represent a complete survey approach when evaluating adult horses with urinary disease. CT in foals would be ideal to guide treatment and provide prognosis in congenital malformation. The use of nuclear scintigraphy and Doppler ultrasound in renal function clinical assessment should be implemented.

DISCLOSURE

The author has nothing to disclose.

SUPPLEMENTARY DATA

Supplementary data related to this article can be found online at doi:10.1016/j.cveq.2021.11.009

REFERENCES

1. Pujol R, De Fourmestraux C, Symoens A, et al. Retroperitoneoscopy in the horse: anatomical study of the retroperitoneal perirenal space and description of a surgical approach. Equine Vet J 2021;53:364–72.
2. Martin LM, Jochems BC, Latmer JC, et al. Idiopathic renal haematuria in an Egyptian Arabian stallion. Equine Vet Educ 2019;31:260–3.
3. Juzwiak JS, Bain FT, Slone DE, et al. Unilateral nephrectomy for treatment of chronic hematuria due to nephrolithiasis in a colt. Can Vet J 1988;29:931–3.
4. Busse NI, Paredes EA, Bustamante HA, et al. Periurethral vascular hamartoma in a 6-month-old foal with idiopathic hematuria: new differential diagnosis. J Equine Vet Sci 2018;67:19–22.
5. Schumacher J, Schumacher J, Schmitz D. Macroscopic haematuria of horses. Equine Vet Educ 2002;14:201–10.
6. Glass KG, Arnold CE, Varner DD, et al. Signalment, clinical features, and outcome for male horses with urethral rents following perineal urethrotomy or corpus spongiotomy: 33 cases (1989–2013). J Am Vet Med Assoc 2016;249:1421–7.

7. Hackett ES, Bruemer J, Hedrickson DA, et al. Buccal mucosal urethroplasty for treatment of recurrent hemospermia in a stallion. J Am Vet Med Assoc 2009;235: 1212–5.

8. Trela JM, Dechant JE, Culp WT, et al. Use of an absorbable urethral stent for the management of a urethral stricture in a stallion. Vet Surg 2016;45:41–8.

9. Trotter GW, Bennett DG, Behm RJ. Urethral calculi in five horses. Vet Surg 1981; 10:159–62.

10. Saam D. Urethrolithiasis and nephrolithiasis in a horse. Can Vet J 2001;42: 880–3.

11. Macbeth BJ. Obstructive urolithiasis, unilateral hydronephrosis, and probable nephrolithiasis in a 12-year old Clydesdale gelding. Can Vet J 2008;49:287–90.

12. Schott HC. Recurrent urolithiasis associated with unilateral pyelonephritis in five equids. Proc Am Assoc Equine Practit 2002;48:136–7.

13. Gosling L, Anderson J, Rendle D. Conservative management of iatrogenic bladder rupture and uroperitoneum in a gelding with urolithiasis. Equine Vet Educ 2021;33:E53–7.

14. Olaiya B, Adler DG. Air embolism secondary to endoscopy in hospitalized patients: results from the National Inpatient Sample (1998-2013). Ann Gastroenterol 2019;32:1–7.

15. Romagnoli N, Rinnovati R, Lukacs RM, et al. Suspected venous air embolism during urinary tract endoscopy in a standing horse. Equine Vet Educ 2014;26: 134–7.

16. Nolen-Walston R. Venous air embolism during cystoscopy in standing horses. Equine Vet Educ 2014;26:138–40.

17. Gordon E, Schlipf JWJ, Husby KA, et al. Two occurrences of presumptive venous air embolism in a gelding during cystoscopy and perineal urethrotomy. Equine Vet Educ 2017;290:236–41.

18. Mirski MA, Lele AV, Fitzsimmons L, et al. Diagnosis and treatment of vascular air embolism. Anesthesiology 2007;106.

19. Abd El Kader NA, Farghali HA, AbuSeida AM, et al. Evaluation of chromocystoscopy in the diagnosis of cystitis in female donkeys. PLoS One 2018;13: E0402596.

20. Rendle DI, Durham AE, Hughes KJ, et al. Long-term management of sabulous cystitis in five horses. Vet Rec 2008;162:783–8.

21. Snalune KL, Mair TS. Peritonitis secondary to necrosis of the apex of the urinary bladder in a post parturient mare. Equine Vet Educ 2006;18:20–6.

22. Keen JA, Pirie RS. Urinary incontinence associated with sabulous urolithiasis: a series of 4 cases. Equine Vet Educ 2006;18:11–9.

23. Rebsamen E, Geyer H, Furst A, et al. Haematuria in two geldings caused by osteochondroma of the os pubis: case reports and anatomic study of the os pubis in 41 cadaveric pelvises. Equine Vet Educ 2012;24:30–7.

24. Saulez MN, Cebra CK, Heidel JR, et al. Encrusted cystitis secondary to *Corynebacterium matruchotii* infection in a horse. J Am Vet Med Assoc 2005;266: 246–8.

25. Reichelt U, Lischer C. Complications associated with transurethral endoscopic-assisted electrohydraulic lithotripsy for treatment of a bladder calculus in a gelding. Equine Vet Educ 2013;25:55–9.

26. Walesby HA, Ragle CA, Booth LC. Laparoscopic repair of ruptured urinary bladder in a stallion. J Am Vet Med Assoc 2002;221:1737–41.

27. Pye JL, Collins NM, Adkins AR. Transurethral endoscopic-guided intraluminal closure of multiple urinary bladder tears in a standing mare. Equine Vet Educ 2018;30:127–31.
28. Schott HC. Urinary incontinence and sabulous urolithiasis: chicken or egg. Equine Vet Educ 2006;18:17–9.
29. Squinas SC, Britton AP. An unusual case of urinary retention and ulcerative cystitis in a horse, sequelae of pelvic abscessation, and adhesions. Can Vet J 2013;54:690–2.
30. Aleman M, Nieto JE, Higgins JK. Ulcerative cystitis associated with phenylbutazone administration in two horses. J Am Vet Med Assoc 2011;239:499–503.
31. Montgomery JB, Duckett WM, Bourque AC. Pelvic lymphoma as a cause of urethral compression in a mare. Can Vet J 2009;50:751–4.
32. Smith FL, Magdesian KG, Michel AO, et al. Equine idiopathic hemorrhagic cystitis: clinical features and comparison with bladder neoplasia. J Vet Intern Med 2018;32:1202–9.
33. Zantigh AJ, Gaughan EM, Bain FT. Squamous cell carcinoma of the urinary bladder in a horse. Compend Continuing Education Veterinarians 2012;34:E1–5.
34. Hurcombe SDA, Slovis NM, Kohn CW, et al. Poorly differentiated leiomyosarcoma of the urogenital tract in a horse. J Am Vet Med Assoc 2008;233:1908–12.
35. Wise LN, Bryan JN, Sellon DC, et al. A retrospective analysis of renal carcinoma in the horse. J Vet Intern Med 2009;23:913–8.
36. Lisowski ZM, Mair TS, Fews D. Transitional cell carcinoma of the urinary bladder in a 12-year-old Belgian warmblood gelding. Equine Vet Educ 2015;27:E20–4.
37. Jones ARE, Ragle CA. A minimally invasive surgical technique for ureteral ostioplasty in two fillies with ureteral ectopia. J Am Vet Med Assoc 2018;253:1467–72.
38. Schott HC, Hdgson DR, Bayly WM. Ureteral catheterisation in the horse. Equine Vet Educ 1990;2:140–3.
39. Strugava L, Dornbulsch LPTC, Silva-Meirelles JR, et al. Catheterization of the renal pelvis guided by cistoscopy in mares. Arq Bras Med Vet Zootec 2018;70:1483–8.
40. Chaney KP. Congenital anomalies of the equine urinary tract. Vet Clin North Am Equine Pract 2007;23:691–6.
41. Sullins KE, McIlwraith CW, Yovich JV, et al. Ectopic ureter managed by unilateral nephrectomy in two female horses. Equine Vet J 1988;20:463–6.
42. Cokelaere SM, Martens A, Vanschandevijl K, et al. Hand-assisted laparoscopic nephrectomy after initial ureterocystostomy in a Shire filly with left ureteral ectopia. Vet Rec 2007;161:424–7.
43. Hahn K, Conze TM, Wollanke B, et al. Urogenital hypoplasia and X chromosome monosomy in a draft horse filly. J Equine Vet Sci 2021;96:103318.
44. Getman LM, Ross W, Elce YA. Bilateral ureterocystostomy to correct left ureteral atresia and right ureteral ectopia in an 8-month-old standardbred filly. Vet Surg 2005;34:657–61.
45. Frederick J, Freeman DE, MacKay RJ, et al. Removal of ureteral calculi in two geldings via a standing flank approach. J Am Vet Med Assoc 2012;241:1214–20.
46. Ferguson N, Couetil L, Hawkins J, et al. Unilateral nephrectomy in two aged horses. Equine Vet Educ 2007;19:300–5.
47. Schott H. Obstructive disease of the urinary tract. Disorders of the urinary system. Equine internal medicine. 4th edition. Maryland Heights, (MD): Elsevier; 2018.

48. Pasquel SG, Agnew D, Nelson N, et al. Ureteropyeloscopic anatomy of the renal pelvis of the horse. Equine Vet J 2013;45:31–8.
49. Trivedi PJ, Braden B. Indications, stains and techniques in chromoendoscopy. Q J Med 2013;106:117–31.
50. Graves EA. Unilateral pyelonephritis in a miniature horse colt. Vet Clin North Am Equine Pract 2006;22:209–17.
51. Matthews HK, Toal RL. A review of equine renal imaging techniques. Vet Radiol Ultrasound 1996;37:163–73.
52. Draper A, Bowel IM, Hallowell GD. Reference ranges and reliability of transabdominal ultrasonographic renal dimensions in thoroughbred horses. Vet Radiol Ultrasound 2012;53:336–41.
53. Reef VB. Adult abdominal ultrasonography. In: Rantanen NW, McKinnon AO, editors. Equine diagnostic ultrasound. Philadelphia, (PA): W. B. Saunders; 1998. p. 273–363.
54. Habershon-Butcher J, Bowen M, Hallowell G. Validation of a novel translumbar ultrasound technique for measuring renal dimensions in horses. Vet Radiol Ultrasound 2014;55:323–30.
55. Diaz O, Smith G, Reef VB. Ultrasonographic appearance of the lower urinary tract in fifteen normal horses. Vet Radiol Ultrasound 2007;48:560–4.
56. Freeman SL. Diagnostic ultrasonography of the mature equine abdomen. Equine Vet Educ 2003;15:319–30.
57. Reis Casiglioni MC, de Campos Vettorato M, Fogaca JL, et al. Quantitative ultrasound of kidneys, liver, and spleen: a comparison between mules and horses. J Equine Vet Sci 2018;70:71–5.
58. Gracia-Calvo LA, Duran ME, Martin-Cuervo M, et al. Persistent hematuria as a result of chronic renal hypertension secondary to nephritis in a stallion. J Equine Vet Sci 2014;34:709–14.
59. Kisthardt KK, Schumacher J, Binn-Bodner ST, et al. Severe renal hemorrhage caused by pyelonephritis in 7 horses: clinical and ultrasonographic evaluation. Can Vet J 1999;40:571–6.
60. Bragato N, Borges NC, Fioravanti MCS. B-mode and Doppler ultrasound of chronic kidney disease in dogs and cats. Vet Res Commun 2017;41:307–15.
61. Macri F, Pugiese M, Di Pietro S, et al. Doppler ultrasonographic estimation of renal resistive index in horse: comparison between left and right kidneys. J Equine Vet Sci 2015;35:111–5.
62. Freccero F, Petrucellil M, Cipone M, et al. Doppler evaluation of renal resistivity index in healthy conscious horses and donkeys. PLoS One 2020;15:E0228741.
63. Siwinska N, Zak A, Slowikowska M, et al. Renal resistive index as a potential indicator of acute kidney injury in horses. J Equine Vet Sci 2021;103:103662.
64. Hilton HG, Aleman M, Maher O, et al. Hand-assisted laparoscopic nephrectomy in a standing horse for the management of renal cell carcinoma. Equine Vet Educ 2008;20:239–44.
65. Barratt-Boyes SM, Spensley M, Nyland TG, et al. Ultrasound localization and guidance for renal biopsy in the horse. Vet Radiol 1991;32:121–6.
66. Ramirez S, Williams J, Seahorn T, et al. Ultrasound-assisted diagnosis of renal dysplasia in a 3-month-old quarter horse colt. Vet Radiol Ultrasound 1998;39:143–4.
67. Tyner GA, Nolen-Walston D, Hall T, et al. A multicenter retrospective study of 151 renal biopsies in horses. J Vet Intern Med 2011;25:532–9.

68. Slovis N. Ultrasonography of the liver, spleen, kidney, bladder, and peritoneal cavity. In: Kidd J,A, Lu KG, Frazer ML, editors. Atlas of equine ultrasonography. Hoboken, (NJ): Wiley-Blackwell, Inc.; 2014. p. 409–26.
69. Hoffmann KL, Wood AKW, McCarthy PH. Ultrasonography of the equine neonatal kidney. Equine Vet J 2000;32:109–13.
70. Beccati F, Lauteri E, Cercone M, et al. Ultrasonographic technique and appearance of adrenal gland in neonatal foals: a pilot study. J Equine Vet Sci 2018; 61:13–7.
71. Sprayberry KA. Ultrasonographic examination of the equine neonate: thorax and abdomen. Vet Clin North Am Equine Pract 2015;31:515–43.
72. Durie I, Van Loon G, Vermeire S, et al. Transrectal ultrasonography of the left adrenal gland in healthy horses. Vet Radiol Ultrasound 2010;51:540–4.
73. Papadopoulos G, Bourdoumi A, Kachrilas S, et al. Hyoscine n-butylbromide (Buscopan®) in the treatment of acute ureteral colic: what is the evidence. Urol Int 2014;92:253–7.
74. Gremillion C, Cohen EB, Vaden S, et al. Optimization of ultrasonographic ureteral jet detection and normal ureteral jet morphology in dogs. Vet Radiol Ultrasound 2021;1–8.
75. Gough SL, Fraser BSL, Rendle DI, et al. Renal dysplasia, ectopic ureter, septic ureterectasia and cryptorchidism in an 11-month-old Cob colt presenting with ascending pyoureter and pyocystis. Equine Vet Educ 2021;33(8):e239–42.
76. Saetra T, Breuhaus B, Hildebran A. Unilateral nephrolithiasis with renal rupture in a horse. Equine Vet Educ 2018;30:635–9.
77. Divers TJ, Whitlock RH. Acute renal failure in six horses resulting from haemodynamic causes. Equine Vet J 1987;19:178–84.
78. Wooldridge AA, Seahorn TL, Williams J, et al. Chronic renal failure associated with nephrolithiasis, ureterolithiasis, and renal dysplasia in a 2-year-old quarter horse gelding. Vet Radiol Ultrasound 1999;40:361–4.
79. Divers TJ, Yeager A. The value of ultrasonographic examination in the diagnosis and management of renal diseases in horses. Equine Vet Educ 1995;7:334–41.
80. Ramirez S, Seahorn TL, Williams J. Renal medullary rim sign in 2 adult quarter horses. Can Vet J 1998;39:647–9.
81. Leveille R, Miyabayashi T, Weisbrode SE, et al. Ultrasonographic renal changes associated with phenylbutazone administration in three foals. Can Vet J 1996; 37:235–6.
82. Blikslager AT, Green EM, MacFadden KE, et al. Excretory urography and ultrasonography in the diagnosis of bilateral ectopic ureters in a foal. Vet Radiol Ultrasound 1992;33:41–7.
83. Rodger LD, Carlson GP, Moran ME, et al. Resolution of a left ureteral stone using electrohydraulic lithotripsy in a thoroughbred colt. J Vet Intern Med 1995;9: 280–2.
84. Abu-Seida AM, Shamaa AA. Ultrasonography and surgical treatment of an unusual case of urethral calculus in an Arabian horse. J Equine Vet Sci 2020;92: 103150.
85. Waldridge BM, Lenz SD, Hudson J, et al. Multiple congenital urogenital abnormalities in a Tennessee walking horse colt. Equine Vet Educ 2009;21:315–8.
86. Gilday RA, Wojnarowicz C, Tryon KA, et al. Bilateral renal dysplasia, hydronephrosis, and hydroureter in a septic neonatal foal. Can Vet J 2015;56:257–60.
87. Gull T, Schmitz DG, Bahr A, et al. Renal hypoplasia and dysplasia in an American miniature foal. Vet Rec 2001;149:199–203.

88. Medina-Torres CE, Hewson J, Stampfli S, et al. Bilateral diffuse cystic renal dysplasia in a 9-day-old thoroughbred filly. Can Vet J 2014;55:141–6.

89. Patterson-Kane JC, Tramontin RR, Giles RCJ, et al. Transitional cell carcinoma of the urinary bladder in a thoroughbred, with intra-abdominal dissemination. Vet Pathol 2000;37:692–5.

90. Serena C, Naranjo C, Koch C, et al. Resection cystoplasty of a squamous cell carcinoma in a mare. Equine Vet Educ 2009;21:263–6.

91. Busechian S, Gialletti R, Brachelente C, et al. Transitional cell carcinoma of the bladder in a 12-year-old gelding. J Equine Vet Sci 2016;40:80–3.

92. Nogradi N, Magdesian KG, Whitcomb MB, et al. Imaging diagnosis: aortic aneurysm and ureteral obstruction secondary to umbilical artery abscessation in a 5-week-old foal. Vet Radiol Ultrasound 2013;54:384–9.

93. Arnold CE, Chaffin MK, Rush BR. Hematuria associated with cystic hematomas in three neonatal foals. J Am Vet Med Assoc 2005;22:778–80.

94. McKenzie HC. Disorders of foals. In: Reed SM, Bayly SM, Sellon DC, editors. Equine internal medicine. 4th edition. Maryland Heights, (MD): Elsevier; 2018. p. 1365–459.

95. Diaz OS, Zarucco L, Dolente B, et al. Sonographic diagnosis of a presumed ureteral tear in a horse. Vet Radiol Ultrasound 2004;45:73–7.

96. Beccati F, Cercone M, Angeli G, et al. Use of multiphase computed tomographic urography in the diagnosis of ureteral tear in a 6-day-old foal. Vet Radiol Ultrasound 2016;57:E10–5.

97. Ferris R, Franklin R, Adams A, et al. Rupture of a penile artery and erectile body. An uncommon cause of dysuria in a horse. Equine Vet Educ 2008;20:564–6.

98. El-Ghar MA, Refaie H, Sharaf D, et al. Diagnosing urinary tract abnormalities: intravenous urography or CT urography. Rep Med Imag 2014;7:55–63.

99. Tomlinson JE, Farnsworth K, Sage AM, et al. Percutaneous ultrasound-guided pyelography aided diagnosis of ectopic ureter and hydronephrosis in a 3-week-old filly. Vet Radiol Ultrasound 2001;42:349–51.

100. Anson A, Strohmayer C, Larrinaga JM, et al. Computed tomographic retrograde positive contrast cystography and computed tomographic excretory urography characterization of a urinary bladder diverticulum in a dog. Vet Radiol Ultrasound 2019;60:E66–70.

101. Coleman MC, Chaffin MK, Arnold CE, et al. The use of computed tomography in the diagnosis of an ectopic ureter in a quarter horse filly. Equine Vet Educ 2011; 23:597–602.

102. Schott HC. Ectopic ureter: a leaky problem no matter how you look at it. Equine Vet Educ 2011;23:603–5.

103. Alexander K, Dunn M, Carmel EN, et al. Clinical application of Patlak plot CT-GFR in animals with upper urinary tract disease. Vet Radiol Ultrasound 2010; 51:421–7.

104. Kang K, Jang M, Choi KU, et al. Antegrade and retrograde CT urethrography with virtual urethroscopy in a dog with urethral narrowing after bilateral triple pelvic osteotomy. Vet Radiol Ultrasound 2019;1–6.

105. Schwarz T, Bommer N, Parys M, et al. Four-dimensional CT excretory urography is an accurate technique for diagnosis of canine ureteral ectopia. Vet Radiol Ultrasound 2021;62:190–8.

106. Hiorns MP. Imaging of the urinary tract: the role of CT and MRI. Pediatr Nephrol 2011;26:59–68.

107. Martin DR, Sharma P, Salman K, et al. Individual kidney blood flow measured with contrast-enhanced first-pass perfusion MR imaging. Radiology 2008;246: 241–8.

108. Matthews HK, Andrews FM, Daniel GB, et al. Comparison of standard and radio-nuclide methods for measurement of glomerular filtration rate and effective renal blood flow in female horses. Am J Vet Res 1992;53:1612–6.

109. Woods P, Drost T, Clarke CR, et al. Use of ^{99m}Tc-mercaptoacetyltriglycine to evaluate renal function in horses. Vet Radiol Ultrasound 2000;41:85–8.

110. Malton R. Nonorthopaedic scintigraphy. In: Dyson SJ, Pilsworth RC, Twardock AR, et al, editors. Equine scintigraphy. Cambridgeshire, UK: Equine Veterinary Journal, Ltd.; 2003. p. 245–9.

Surgery of the Equine Urinary Tract

Susan L. Fubini, DVM*, Michelle Delco, DVM, PhD

KEYWORDS

- Uroabdomen • Urolithiasis • Ectopic ureter • Nephrectomy • Urethra

KEY POINTS

- Careful and complete perioperative care is essential to successful urinary surgery in the horse.
- Sophisticated endoscopic and imaging capabilities may be necessary for determination of the appropriate surgical procedure.
- Laparoscopy is becoming more commonplace in urinary surgery.
- Some procedures, such as ruptured urinary bladder repair, may seem straightforward, but can be complicated by involvement of other, related structures.

This article provides an overview of surgical procedures of the urinary tract in foals and horses. Although some of the procedures described require general anesthesia and a surgical suite, there may be options, in some instances, to do the surgery in the standing, sedated horse. With appropriate perioperative case management favorable outcomes are expected. A large number of references are provided for further surgical detail.

Uroperitoneum in foals is usually treated surgically. A discussion of clinical signs, clinical pathology findings, and medical management is provided elsewhere in this issue. Most commonly, uroperitoneum is a result of urinary bladder rupture following parturition in colts.[1–4] A persistent, patent, or urachal rent can also cause uroperitoneum,[3,5–8] and rarely, ureteral defects.[6,9–13] Typically, urinary bladder defects are located dorsally and are 2 to 5 cm in length. The edges of the tear vary in appearance, from irregular to inflamed and smooth (**Fig. 1**). Ultrasound of the umbilicus and associated structures is helpful to determine the extent of the pathology.[14,15] Rupture of the urinary bladder in adult horses is rare but has been reported following outflow obstruction of the urinary tract, trauma, previous surgery, and rarely following parturition.[16–22]

Once medically stabilized, the patient is placed under general anesthesia in dorsal recumbency. The caudal abdomen is prepared for aseptic surgery. The umbilicus should be cleaned and, if inflamed, oversewn with a continuous suture. The surgeon may elect to place an indwelling urinary catheter by passing an appropriately sized

Department of Clinical Sciences, Cornell University, Ithaca, NY 14853
* Corresponding Author.
E-mail address: slf3@cornell.edu

Vet Clin Equine 38 (2022) 141–153
https://doi.org/10.1016/j.cveq.2021.11.010
0749-0739/22/© 2021 Elsevier Inc. All rights reserved.

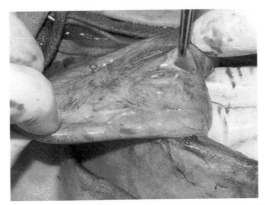

Fig. 1. Tear along the dorsal aspect of the urinary bladder in a 3-day-old male foal.

stallion catheter retrograde from the penile urethra and suturing the aseptically prepared preputial orifice around the catheter to keep it in place during surgery. The end of the catheter is attached to a fluid bag, making a closed system. The area is draped off before surgery, and a sharp, fusiform incision is made around the umbilicus and extended caudad. In colts, the skin incision is extended caudally 2 to 3 cm lateral to ventral midline to avoid the prepuce. The incision is continued through the subcutaneous tissues, external rectus sheath, bluntly through the rectus muscle and then the internal rectus sheath and peritoneum are tented and incised. Alternatively, the penis and prepuce are reflected to the side and the body wall incision continued on ventral midline through the subcutaneous tissues, and linea alba. Entry into the abdomen should be done carefully and preferably on the lateral side of the incision, away from the umbilical remnants that run along the ventral midline, if they persist. This includes the round ligament of the liver (remnant of the umbilical vein) coursing cranially, and the urachus and lateral ligaments of the urinary bladder (remnants of the umbilical arteries) traveling caudally from the umbilicus and along the lateral margins of the urinary bladder. It is often necessary to identify the umbilical remnants and ligate them. At this stage, a defect in the urachus or urinary bladder would be apparent (**Fig. 2**). If a defect in the urinary bladder is not readily identifiable, distending the

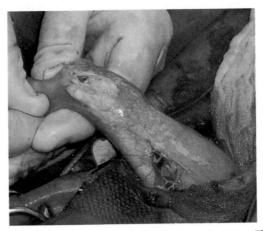

Fig. 2. Urachal rupture in a foal that presented with uroperitoneum. The umbilical artery remnant is enlarged.

bladder with saline or a dilute solution of methylene blue or fluorescein dye via the urinary catheter may help to demonstrate the rent. Occasionally, ventral tears occur and tend to travel toward the neck of the urinary bladder.[23] Once the defect is identified it is helpful to apply stay sutures on either side of the tear, pack off the abdomen, and have fluid suction ready. The urinary bladder is closed in two layers using 2–0 or 3–0 monofilament absorbable suture. The second layer should be an inverting pattern. Historically veterinary surgeons have avoided sutures that penetrate the mucosa to avoid potential nidus formation; however, with the advent of inert, synthetic, monofilament suture this may be less of a concern. Some advocate debriding the edges of the defect, but with an inverted closure this is not needed. It may be necessary to extend the incision caudad if additional exposure is required to ligate and resect the umbilical artery remnants.

Alternatively, laparoscopy can be used to assist resection of umbilical structures in foals.[24] Laparoscopy has also been used for urinary bladder repair in foals.[25]

In the adult horse exposure to the urinary bladder is limited. Furthermore, tears tend to be deeper at the neck of the bladder.[20,23] Options for surgical access include a caudal paramedian approach under general anesthesia. Standing approaches have also been described. In mares several authors have successfully everted the urinary bladder through the urethral sphincter (with and without a sphincterotomy).[16,20,21,26] Complications include urine scalding and delayed vaginal wound healing. Laparoscopy is another option, although visualization maybe difficult in a recently foaled mare and there is a learning curve for the operator.[27–29] There are two recent reports of successfully repairing tears in a standing mare using minimally invasive techniques with direct suturing,[30] or an endoscopic suturing device.[31]

Conservative management has been reported for tears that would be difficult to approach surgically.[32] Typically, a Foley catheter is maintained in the urinary bladder for decompression. In males this is via perineal urethrotomy (PU). The animal is stabilized with intravenous fluids and electrolyte abnormalities corrected. Peritoneal dialysis helps to control elevated serum urea nitrogen and creatinine values and keep electrolyte balance. Reports by Peitzmeier and Slone[33] and Gosling and coworkers[34] suggest resolution can occur by 14 days following placement of an indwelling catheter.

If uroperitoneum is secondary to a patent urachus, the procedure is similar to the above description. A fusiform incision is made around the umbilicus, and the dissection is continued through subcutaneous tissues, external rectus sheath, rectus muscle, and internal rectus sheath and peritoneum. The umbilical remnants are ligated and the apex of the urinary bladder is resected, as described previously.[23] Urachal defects can leak urine intra-abdominally and/or into the subcutaneous tissues (**Fig. 3**), and the presence of considerable preputial swelling should increase the suspicion of a urachal tear. The diagnosis is made by clinical findings alone but measuring serum urea nitrogen and creatinine on fluid aspirated from the swelling is confirmatory.[35] Although the tissue is not ideal for surgical repair, the continued accumulation of subcutaneous urine can result in straining on the part of the foal and necrosis of the involved tissues. Medical management with an indwelling urinary catheter, parenteral antibiotics, and anti-inflammatory medications are used, but surgical repair is definitive. It may be necessary to keep a drain in place for 48 to 72 hours postoperatively.

Defects in the ureter causing retroperitoneal accumulation of urine or uroperitoneum are much less common but have been reported in male and female foals of various breeds.[2,6,9–13] These animals tended to be several days older than those with urachal or urinary bladder lesions, typically presenting at 4 to 16 days of age. Cause of this condition remains speculative, but may be congenital and/or traumatic.

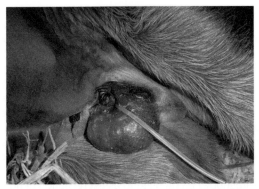

Fig. 3. Subcutaneous accumulation of urine in a foal with a urachal rupture. A urinary catheter is in place.

Ureteral defects are single or multiple, complicating the repair. The diagnosis of a ureteral tear is most often made (and should be suspected) when animals are being explored for uroperitoneum and no lesions are identified in the urinary bladder or urachus. Additional diagnostic procedures may be needed to define the site of the tear.[36] Cystoscopy with catheterization of the ureters and injection of a dye, such as methylene blue, may allow for demonstration of a ureteral rent. The use of ultrasound may be helpful and more advanced imaging, such as an intravenous pyelogram and multiphase computed tomographic urography, can also be diagnostic.[37] Primary repair of these defects using small (5–0) suture with and without a stent has been reported, as has unilateral nephrectomy to treat affected animals.[37] Ureteral defects in adult horses are extremely rare but have been reported following abdominal trauma.[36,38,39] Two animals were treated conservatively and one had a stent placed; all survived.

SURGERY FOR UROLITHIASIS

The incidence of equine urolithiases seems to vary widely based on geographic location. Uroliths most commonly occur in the bladder, but may also be present in the ureter, urethra, and kidney.[40] In a study by Laverty in 1992 the authors documented the anatomic location of uroliths in 68 horses: urinary bladder (n = 47), urethra (n = 11) **(Fig. 4)**, kidneys (n = 15), and ureter (n = 2).[40] Affected horses typically present with stranguria, pollakiuria, and/or hematuria.[23,] Diagnosis is based on rectal examination, ultrasound, and cystoscopy.[38] The clinician must be aware that on rectal examination, it is possible to miss a stone in a distended urinary bladder, and, therefore, should be prepared to pass a urinary catheter to empty urine from the bladder. Stones have typically been classified into types I and II. Both are made up of primarily calcium carbonate. Type I stones are usually ovoid, yellow-green in color, and spiculated **(Fig. 5)**. They are sometimes, but not always, easy to fragment. Type II stones are less common, more irregular in shape, have a smooth contour **(Fig. 6)**, and contain more phosphate than type I. When the stones are sectioned and imaged, irregular concentric bands are evident around a central core. There are small areas filled with crystalline material, which may explain the porosity of some of the uroliths. Ultrasound examination of the kidneys should be performed in horses with cystic or urethral calculi to rule out nephrolithiasis, hydronephrosis, and to assess the likelihood of recurrence.

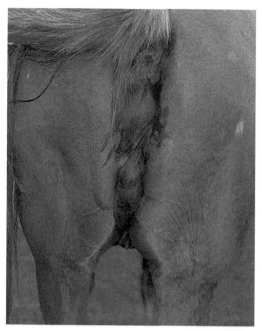

Fig. 4. Large urethral urolith evident in a gelding presented for anuria.

There are many reported approaches to address cystic calculi. These include laparoscopic procedures, celiotomies, perineal approaches, and a variety of lithotripsy procedures.[23,41–55] Historically, celiotomy approaches were used most commonly. These included caudal ventral midline for mares and a paramedian or a caudal parainguinal celiotomy for geldings and stallions.[23,43,53,55] For the latter, the incision is continued as a paramedian or parainguinal celiotomy, or the penis and prepuce is reflected, and the incision into the abdomen made on ventral midline. The urinary

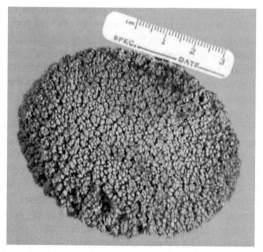

Fig. 5. Type I urolith retrieved from the urinary bladder of an adult horse.

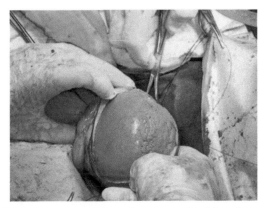

Fig. 6. Type II urolith being removed from the urinary bladder of an adult horse during laprocystotomy.

bladder is difficult to exteriorize, resulting in several reports documenting ways to improve access. These include dilating the urinary bladder with sterile saline and/or lidocaine and wrapping a large laparotomy sponge around the bladder neck to hold it in place.[54] One report suggests making a caudal midline approach large enough for the surgeon to insert an arm, locate the calculus, and elevate it to the body wall while another surgeon makes a second celiotomy, just large enough to manipulate the calculus to the outside for removal.[55] The second, small, incision helps to prevent retraction of the urinary bladder into the abdomen. In the author's experience these approaches are useful, but are more difficult in overconditioned individuals, because access to the abdomen is reduced with the extra body wall thickness.

A perirectal approach has also been described in the standing animal using Gokel cystotomy.[56] This procedure is performed with intravenous sedation, epidural anesthesia, and a perirectal incision to gain access to the urinary bladder. A 15-cm sharp incision is made in the perirectal space and blunt dissection is used to approach the urinary bladder. The trigone region of the bladder is located and the internal pudendal artery, vein, and nerve are identified and avoided. The calculus is retracted and stabilized in the neck of the bladder. Concurrent cystoscopy is useful in confirming the location of the ureters and guiding incision placement over the calculus. A 2-cm sharp incision is made over the calculus and the cystotomy incision is digitally enlarged, if necessary, to facilitate calculus removal. If desired, the cystotomy incision is closed primarily or it can be left to heal via second intention with an indwelling catheter.

Other options in the standing horse include a temporary PU in males or transurethral manipulation in females using sedation and epidural anesthesia. These are the techniques used most commonly in the author's hospital. In males, a stallion catheter is placed in the urethra from the penis in retrograde fashion. A 10-cm sharp incision is made 5 to 10 cm ventral to the anus, centered over the palpable ischial arch. A combination of blunt and sharp dissection is used to continue the dissection on midline down to the urethral catheter. The urethra is incised and the stallion catheter retracted to the ventral extent of the surgical site, allowing access to the urinary bladder but preventing debris from becoming lodged in the subischial urethra. Techniques used to manipulate the calculus, or break them up if they are very large, include manual crushing with an instrument or jack hammer, fragmentation with a mallet and osteotome, pulsed-dye laser, holmium:yttrium-aluminum-garnet laser, and electrohydraulic or ballistic shockwave.[44–49,51,52,57,58] A laparoscopic retrieval bag is passed through the urethral orifice in mares or via the PU in male animals. The calculus is located per rectum with one hand, which is used to manipulate the stone into the bag. In mares it is sometimes possible for a surgeon with a small hand to manually dilate the urethral sphincter, insert a hand into the bladder, and manipulate the calculus into a retrieval bag.[44,57] Large Endocatch bags are ideal for this purpose, but it is also possible to use a sturdy bag, such as a sterile radiograph cassette holder. The lip of the bag is then drawn out of the urethra or urethrotomy circumferentially, and traction is placed on the bag to exteriorize and remove smaller stones. For large calculi, the bag is used to retain and retract the calculus caudally so that it may be broken up with one of the techniques mentioned. Another option in the mare is to perform a longitudinal sphincterotomy to improve access to the lumen of the urinary bladder.[23] The urinary bladder should be copiously lavaged to remove any sediment or fragments that remain. If performed, the sphincterotomy is closed routinely. The PU is left open to heal by second intention. The horse should be monitored for recurrence.

Ureterotomy has been performed via a flank celiotomy to remove ureteroliths.[59] The authors in a 2012 paper[59] describe being able to mobilize the ureter and exteriorize it through a flank incision. The calculus could not be moved within the lumen of the ureter necessitating an ureterotomy approximately 25 cm proximal to the calculus, which was fragmented using a uterine biopsy forceps and removed. The ureter was lavaged and closed.

To prevent urolith formation it is recommended to decrease the calcium intake by feeding less alfalfa hay and/or installing water softening filtration systems on farms with hard water. Additionally, feed is salted to encourage water intake. Attempts have been made to alter the pH of the equine urine to help to prevent the formation of calcium carbonate uroliths using an anionic dietary supplement to achieve feed with a very low dietary cation-anion difference.[60] Although this feeding regimen did lower the urine pH it was not sufficiently low to prevent urolith formation. Furthermore, the palatability of the feed was problematic.

ECTOPIC URETER

Ureteral ectopia is a rare developmental anomaly in horses.[36] No breed predilection has been confirmed but most reported cases are in quarter horses and standardbreds.[36] Affected animals can have unilateral or bilateral involvement. Presenting signs include urinary incontinence, urine scald, pollakiuria, and/or dribbling urine. The opening of the aberrant ureters is located at various sites along the urogenital tract, including the neck of the bladder or urethra, and can sometimes be visualized in fillies during vaginoscopy. Cystoscopic examination can often confirm the diagnosis; in unilateral cases only one ureteral opening is found, and the ectopic ureter may be seen coursing along the dorsal bladder wall without an opening into the bladder. The use of a dye, such as phenolsulfonphthalein (phenol red) at 0.01 mg/kg intravenously, can color the urine and aid in identification of the abnormal opening.[36] Retrograde ureterography has been used with catheterization of the urinary bladder and ureters, as have antegrade studies via ultrasound-guided pyelography,[61,62] and excretory urography and ultrasonography[63]; however, it is difficult to achieve sufficient detail. With foals or miniature horses, imaging using computed tomography with contrast or MRI may provide definitive information; however, these modalities require general anesthesia and are costly.[64]

Traditionally, ectopic ureters have been treated by ureterocystostomy[61,65,66] or unilateral nephrectomy.[67–69] Before surgery it is essential to determine if the condition is unilateral or bilateral, which side is affected, whether infection is present, and the status of the renal function. Ultrasonography of both ureters and kidneys is helpful in confirming the affected sides, because fillies with ectopic ureter often have concurrent ipsilateral ureteral distention. To rule out detrusor and urethral sphincter dysfunction, saline is infused into the urinary bladder to ensure fluid is voided normally.

Ureterocystostomy has been successful, but is difficult if the ureter is enlarged and distorted. If the condition is unilateral and the ureter is abnormal, or a urinary tract infection (which is common in fillies 4 weeks or older) or unilateral hydronephrosis is present, a unilateral nephrectomy may be the best option (see later). A novel approach to ectopic ureter was described in 2018 by Jones and Ragle.[70] Standing ureteral ostioplasty was performed via cystoscopy in two fillies at 1 and 3 months of age. The urethra and urinary bladder were distended with air. A laparoscopic scissor or vessel sealing device (Ligasure) was inserted into the ectopic ureteral ostium, located in the urethra. A longitudinal incision was made, starting at ureteral ostium and extending cranially along the intramural portion of the ureter, to approximately the level of the normal ureteral opening into the bladder. The outcome was favorable in both animals.

NEPHRECTOMY

The main reasons for performing a unilateral nephrectomy include ectopic ureter, renal trauma, infection, nephrolithiasis, neoplasia, parasitism, and idiopathic renal hematuria.[36,67–69,71–73] When a procedure is difficult there are often many ways that it is done and that is the case with nephrectomy. Abdominal approaches include standing through a flank approach with a rib resection, usually the 16th or 17th (right side) or 17th or 18th (left side) or a similar incision under general anesthesia. Horses have also been anesthetized and positioned in a standing position against a tilt table to allow for the advantages of a standing approach while the animal is immobilized. Postoperative myopathy is a risk of this technique. A ventral midline incision has been used for foals[36] and more recently described in adult horses.[67] Hand-assisted laparoscopic and laparoscopic removal[68,74] also have been used. If the animal is anesthetized positive pressure ventilation should be available because it is possible to enter the thoracic cavity.

Regardless of positioning if a rib resection is used a sharp incision made directly over the rib and extend for 30 to 40 cm. The musculature is incised as is the periosteum. The periosteum is elevated at the site of the rib transection proximally, avoiding the intercostal vasculature that runs along the caudal border of the rib. The rib is transected proximally with Gigli wire, or a bone saw, and disarticulated distally at the costochondral junction. The perirenal fat is dissected, mostly bluntly, to identify the renal vasculature and ureter. Smaller capsular vessels and accessory arteries are ligated or controlled with cautery or a vessel sealing device. The renal artery and vein are double ligated individually. As much of the ureter as possible is removed after ligation. The site is checked for hemorrhage, and lavaged copiously, especially if the kidney was infected. It may be appropriate to place a Penrose or other drain if there is considerable dead space. The periosteum and deep fascia are closed followed by subcutaneous tissues and skin.

Laparoscopic and hand-assisted laparoscopic nephrectomy have been described.[68,74,75] To facilitate surgical manipulation during laparoscopy, it may be beneficial to decrease abdominal fill by restricting hay intake for 48 hours before surgery, and/or to induce splenic contraction intraoperatively with phenylephrine (for the left side). At least three portals are used, and the animals are sedated in standing stocks. Regional local anesthesia is employed. Some insufflation (intra-abdominal pressure of 4 mm Hg) is used.[69] From here the procedure is done with laparoscopic instrumentation[74] or with a minilaparotomy and hand assisted.[69] The former requires some specialized laparoscopic ligation instruments and intrarenal anesthesia. The hand-assisted technique permits easier circumferential isolation and mobilization of the kidney.[69]

As minimally invasive techniques continue to be investigated in equine surgery new skills are required and a more thorough anatomic understanding of body cavities is essential. To that end an anatomic study of the retroperitoneal perirenal space was published recently.[73] This work provides anatomic landmarks to help perfect retroperitoneal renal surgery.

SURGERY OF THE URETHRA

Defects in the urethral mucosa in the form of a tear or rupture has been recognized in geldings and stallions and can result in hemospermia and/or hematuria. These lesions usually appear as linear in orientation and extend into the corpus spongiosum (CS) at the level of the ischial arch, on the convex surface of the urethra.[50,76–78] The diagnosis should be suspected with the presenting complaint of hemospermia or hematuria occurring only at the completion of urination, and can usually be confirmed on urethroscopy. How these defects originate is not clear, but is speculated to be the result of increased pressure in this area, where the urethra is fairly narrow, during urination and/or ejaculation.[77,79] Treatment is aimed at decreasing this pressure by performing either a PU or a similar incision that extends to the level of the CS but not through the urethral mucosa. If this is unsuccessful, there are reports of direct suturing of the defect via a PU with urethroscopic assistance,[79] laser application to the edges of the defect combined with perineal surgery,[50] and repair of the lesion using a buccal mucosal graft.[80] There is also a description of using topical 4% policresulen solution infused via retrograde catheterization of the urethra to the level of the ischial arch to essentially chemically cauterize the lesion.[81] The treatment consisted of 100 mL of the solution infused every 48 hours for a total of four to seven treatments with excellent results. As is likely true for any technique, the authors caution that sexual rest was essential for success.

The perineal surgery is done in the standing sedated animal using regional and/or epidural anesthesia. A sterile stallion urinary catheter is placed aseptically in retrograde fashion past the ischial arch. A sharp, approximately 7-cm incision is made on midline 4 to 5 cm distal to the anus. The incision is deepened creating a plane of dissection between the paired retractor penis muscles, the bulbospongiosus muscle, and through the tunica albuginea of the CS. During dissection, the surgeon palpates the urinary catheter to maintain the correct orientation. The CS is incised and, although the incision can be continued through the urethral mucosa, this does not seem to be necessary because decompressing the cavernous tissue presumably provides the pressure dissipation required for the rent to heal.[79] Urine scalding is a complication that is typically temporary, but does require cleaning and application of an emollient daily. Stricture is also a concern but is more common a problem in the distal urethra.[82] Recurrence is an issue and further surgery may be required.

DISCLOSURE

The authors have nothing to disclose.

REFERENCES

1. Rooney JR. Rupture of the urinary bladder in the foal. Vet Pathol 1971;8:445–51.
2. Richardson DW, Kohn CW. Uroperitoneum in the foal. J Am Vet Med Assoc 1983; 182:267–71.

3. Hackett RP. Rupture of the urinary bladder in neonatal foals. Comp Cont Educ Pract Vet 1984;6:5448–54.

4. Hardy J. Uroperitoneum in foals. Equine Vet Educ 1998;10:21–5.

5. Adams R, Koterba AM, Cudd TC, et al. Exploratory celiotomy for suspected urinary tract disruption in neonatal foals: a review of 18 cases. Equine Vet J 1988; 20:3–17.

6. Robertson JT, Spurlock GH, Bramlage LL, et al. Repair of ureteral defect in a foal. J Am Vet Med Assoc 1983;183:799–800.

7. Kablack KA, Embertson RM, Bernard WV, et al. Uroperitoneum in the hospitalised equine neonate: retrospective study of 31 cases, 1988-1997. Equine Vet J 2000; 32:505–8.

8. Dunkel B, Palmer JE, Olson KN, et al. Uroperitoneum in 32 foals: influence of intravenous fluid therapy, infection, and sepsis. J Vet Intern Med 2005;19:889–93.

9. Stickle RL, Wilcock BP, Huseman JL. Multiple ureteral defects in a Belgian foal. Vet Med Small Anim Clin 1975;70:819–21.

10. Divers TJ, Byars TD, Spirito M. Correction of bilateral ureteral defects in a foal. J Am Vet Med Assoc 1988;192:384–6.

11. Cutler TJ, Mackay RJ, Johnson CM, et al. Bilateral ureteral tears in a foal. Aust Vet J 1997;75:413–5.

12. Jean D, Marcoux M, Louf CF. Congenital bilateral distal defect of the ureters in a foal. Equine Vet Educ 1998;10:17–20.

13. Morisset SF, Hawkins J, Frank N, et al. Surgical management of a ureteral defect with ureterorrhaphy and of ureteritis with ureteroneocystostomy in a foal. J Am Vet Med Assoc 2002;220:354–8.

14. Reef VB, Collatos C, Spencer PA, et al. Clinical, ultrasonographic, and surgical findings in foals with umbilical remnant infections. J Am Vet Med Assoc 1989; 195:69–72.

15. Reef VB, Collatos C. Ultrasonography of umbilical structures in clinically normal foals. Am J Vet Res 1988;49:2143–6.

16. White KK. Urethral sphincterotomy as an approach to repair of rupture of the urinary bladder in the mare: a case report. J Equine Med Surg 1977;1:250–3.

17. Nyrop KA, DeBowes RM, Cox JH, et al. Rupture of the urinary bladder in two postparturient mares. Comp Cont Educ Pract Vet 1985;60:S51–513.

18. Tulleners EP, Richardson DW, Reid BV. Vaginal evisceration of the small intestine in three mares. J Am Vet Med Assoc 1985;186:385–7.

19. Jones PA, Sertich PS, Johnston JK. Uroperitoneum associated with ruptured urinary bladder in a postpartum mare. Aust Vet J 1996;74:354–8.

20. Rodgerson DH, Spirito MA, Thorpe PE, et al. Standing surgical repair of cystorrhexis in two mares. Vet Surg 1999;28:113–6.

21. Higuchi T, Nanao Y, Senba H. Repair of urinary bladder rupture through a urethrotomy and urethral sphincterotomy in four postpartum mares. Vet Surg 2002; 31:344–8.

22. Pankowski RL, Fubini SL. Urinary bladder rupture in a two-year-old horse: sequel to a surgically repaired neonatal injury. J Am Vet Med Assoc 1987;191:560–2.

23. Schott H, Woodie J. Bladder. In: Auer J, Stick JA, Kummerle J, et al, editors. Equine surgery. Maryland Heights, (MD): Elsevier; 2019. p. 1129.

24. Fischer ATJ. Laparoscopically assisted resection of umbilical structures in foals. J Am Vet Med Assoc 1999;214:1813–6.

25. Edwards RB, Ducharme NG, Hackett RP. Laparoscopic repair of a bladder rupture in a foal. Vet Surg 1995;24:60–3.

26. Stephen JO, Harty MS, Hollis AR, et al. A non-invasive technique for standing surgical repair of urinary bladder rupture in a post-partum mare: a case report. Ir Vet J 2009;62:734–6.

27. Hendrickson DA, Wilson DG. Instrumentation and techniques for laparoscopic and thoracoscopic surgery in the horse. Vet Clin North Am Equine Pract 1996; 12:235–59.

28. Tuohy JL, Hendrickson DA, Hendrix SM, et al. Standing laparoscopic repair of a ruptured urinary bladder in a mature draught horse. Equine Vet Educ 2009;21: 257–61.

29. Walesby HA, Ragle CA, Booth LC. Laparoscopic repair of ruptured urinary bladder in a stallion. J Am Vet Med Assoc 2002;221:1737–41.

30. Hall MD, Rodgerson DH. Transurethral intraluminal closure of a caudally located bladder neck tear in a standing mare. Equine Vet Educ 2019;32:E111–5.

31. Pye JL, Collins NM, Adkins AR. Transurethral endoscopic-guided intraluminal closure of multiple urinary bladder tears in a standing mare. Equine Vet Educ 2018;30:127–31.

32. Gibson KT, Trotter GW, Gustafson SB, et al. Conservative management of uroperitoneum in a gelding. J Am Vet Med Assoc 1992;200:1692–4.

33. Peitzmeier MD, Slone DE. Management of bladder rupture in mature horses. Equine Vet Educ 2019;33:122–3.

34. Gosling L, Anderson J, Rendle D. Conservative management of iatrogenic bladder rupture and uroperitoneum in a gelding with urolithiasis. Equine Vet Educ 2019;33:E53–7.

35. Lees MJ, Easley KJ, Sutherland RJ, et al. Subcutaneous rupture of the urachus, its diagnosis and surgical management in three foals. Equine Vet J 1989;21: 462–4.

36. Schott H, Woodie J. Kidneys and ureter. In: Auer J, Stick JA, Kummerle J, et al, editors. Equine surgery. 5TH ed. Maryland Heights, (MD): Elsevier; 2009. p. 1115.

37. Beccati F, Cercone M, Angeli G, et al. Imaging diagnosis: use of multiphase computed tomographic urography in the diagnosis of ureteral tear in a 6-day-old foal. Vet Radiol Ultrasound 2016;57:E10–5.

38. Diaz OS, Zarucco L, Dolente B, et al. Sonographic diagnosis of a presumed ureteral tear in a horse. Vet Radiol Ultrasound 2004;45:73–7.

39. Voss ED, Taylor DS, Slovis NM. Use of a temporary indwelling ureteral stent catheter in a mare with a traumatic ureteral tear. J Am Vet Med Assoc 1999;214: 1523–6.

40. Laverty S, Pascoe JR, Ling GV, et al. Urolithiasis in 68 horses. Vet Surg 1992;21: 56–62.

41. Holt PE, Pearson H. Urolithiasis in the horse: a review of 13 cases. Equine Vet J 1984;16:31–4.

42. Lowe JE. Suprapubic cystotomy in a gelding. Cornell Vet 1960;50:510–4.

43. Lowe JE. Surgical removal of equine uroliths via the laparocystotomy approach. J Am Vet Med Assoc 1961;139:345–8.

44. Williamson AJ, McKinnon AO. Transurethral removal of a cystic urolith in a mare using a laparoscopic specimen pouch. Aust Vet J 2017;95:1174–7.

45. Ragle CA. Dorsally recumbent urinary endoscopic surgery. Vet Clin North Am Equine Pract 2000;16:343–50.

46. Straticò P, Suriano R, Sciarrini C, et al. Laparoscopic-assisted cystotomy and cystostomy for treatment of cystic calculus in a gelding. Vet Surg 2012;41:634–7.

47. Röcken M, Stehle C, Mosel G, et al. Laparoscopic-assisted cystotomy for urolith removal in geldings. Vet Surg 2006;35:394–7.
48. Howard RD, Pleasant RS, May KA. Pulsed dye laser lithotripsy for treatment of urolithiasis in two geldings. J Am Vet Med Assoc 1998;212:1600–3.
49. Judy CE, Galuppo LD. Endoscopic-assisted disruption of urinary calculi using a holmium:YAG laser in standing horses. Vet Surg 2002;31:245–50.
50. Madron M, Schleining M, Caston S, et al. Laser treatment of urethral defects in geldings and stallions used as the primary treatment or in combination with a temporary subischial incision: eight cases (2003-2011). Equine Vet Educ 2013; 25:368–73.
51. Röcken M, Fürst A, Kummer M, et al. Endoscopic-assisted electrohydraulic shockwave lithotripsy in standing sedated horses. Vet Surg 2012;41:620–4.
52. Grant DC, Westropp JL, Shiraki R, et al. Holmium:YAG laser lithotripsy for urolithiasis in horses. J Vet Intern Med 2009;23:1079–85.
53. Beard W. Parainguinal laparocystotomy for urolith removal in geldings. Vet Surg 2004;33:386–90.
54. Russell T, Pollock PJ. Local anesthesia and hydro-distension to facilitate cystic calculus removal in horses. Vet Surg 2012;41:638–42.
55. Watts AE, Fubini SL. Modified parainguinal approach for cystic calculus removal in five equids. Equine Vet J 2013;45:94–6.
56. Abuja GA, García-López JM, Doran R, et al. Pararectal cystotomy for urolith removal in nine horses. Vet Surg 2010;39:654–9.
57. Katzman SA, Vaughan B, Nieto JE, et al. Use of a laparoscopic specimen retrieval pouch to facilitate removal of intact or fragmented cystic calculi from standing sedated horses: 8 cases (2012–2015). J Am Vet Med Assoc 2016;249:304–10.
58. May KA, Pleasant RS, Howard RD. Failure of holmium:yttrium-aluminum-garnet laser lithotripsy in two horses with calculi in the urinary bladder. J Am Vet Med Assoc 2001;219:957–61.
59. Frederick J, Freeman DE, Mackay RJ, et al. Removal of ureteral calculi in two geldings via a standing flank approach. J Am Vet Med Assoc 2012;241:1214–20.
60. Nelson EA, Sanchez LC, Mallicote MF, et al. Effect of a commercial anionic dietary supplement on urinary pH and concentrations of electrolytes and pH in blood of horses. N Z Vet J 2020;68:60–4.
61. Pringle JK, Ducharme NG, Baird JD. Ectopic ureter in the horse: three cases and a review of the literature. Can Vet J 1990;31:26–30.
62. Tomlinson JE, Farnsworth K, Sage AM, et al. Percutaneous ultrasound-guided pyelography aided diagnosis of ectopic ureter and hydronephrosis in a 3-week-old filly. Vet Radiol Ultrasound 2001;42:349–51.
63. Blikslager AT, Green EM, MacFadden KE, et al. Excretory urography and ultrasonography in the diagnosis of bilateral ectopic ureters in a foal. Vet Radiol Ultrasound 1992;33:41–7.
64. Coleman MC, Chaffin MK, Arnold CE, et al. The use of computed tomography in the diagnosis of an ectopic ureter in a Quarter Horse filly. Equine Vet Educ 2011; 32:597–602.
65. Getman LM, Ross MW, Elce YA. Bilateral ureterocystostomy to correct left ureteral atresia and right ureteral ectopia in an 8-month-old standardbred filly. Vet Surg 2005;34:657–61.
66. Squire KR, Adams SG. Bilateral ureterocystostomy in a 450-kg horse with ectopic ureters. J Am Vet Med Assoc 1992;201:1213–5.
67. Arnold CE, Taylor T, Chaffin MK, et al. Nephrectomy via ventral median celiotomy in equids. Vet Surg 2013;42:275–9.

68. Keoughan CG, Rodgerson DH, Brown MP. Hand-assisted laparoscopic left nephrectomy in standing horses. Vet Surg 2003;32:206–12.

69. Röcken M, Mosel G, Stehle C, et al. Left- and right-sided laparoscopic-assisted nephrectomy in standing horses with unilateral renal disease. Vet Surg 2007;36: 568–72.

70. Jones ARE, Ragle CA. A minimally invasive surgical technique for ureteral ostioplasty in two fillies with ureteral ectopia. J Am Vet Med Assoc 2018;253:1467–71.

71. Mitchell KJ, Dowling BA, Hughes KJ, et al. Unilateral nephrectomy as a treatment for renal trauma in a foal. Aust Vet J 2004;82:753–5.

72. Sullins KE, Mcilwraith CW, Yovich JV, et al. Ectopic ureter managed by unilateral nephrectomy in two female horses. Equine Vet J 1988;20:463–6.

73. Pujol R, De Fourmestraux C, Symoens A, et al. Retroperitoneoscopy in the horse: anatomical study of the retroperitoneal perirenal space and description of a surgical approach. Equine Vet J 2021;3:364–72.

74. Marien T. Laparoscopic nephrectomy in the standing horse. In: Fischer AT, editor. Equine diagnostic and surgical laparoscopy. Philadelphia, (PA): W. B. Saunders; 2002. p. 273–6.

75. Cokelaere SM, Martens A, Vanschandevjil K, et al. Hand-assisted laparoscopic nephrectomy after initial ureterocystostomy in a Shire filly with left ureteral ectopia. Vet Rec 2007;161:424–7.

76. Lloyd KC, Wheat JD, Ryan AM, et al. Ulceration in the proximal portion of the urethra as a cause of hematuria in horses: four cases (1978-1985). J Am Vet Med Assoc 1989;194:1324–6.

77. Schumacher J, Varner DD, Schmitz DG, et al. Urethral defects in geldings with hematuria and stallions with hemospermia. Vet Surg 1995;24:250–4.

78. Hackett RP, Vaughan JT, Tennant BC. The urinary system [kidneys, urinary bladder, urethra, diseases, horses]. 3rd edition. St. Louis, Missouri: American Veterinary Publications; 1983.

79. Glass KG, Arnold CE, Varner DD, et al. Signalment, clinical features, and outcome for male horses with urethral rents following perineal urethrotomy or corpus spongiotomy: 33 cases (1989-2013). J Am Vet Med Assoc 2016;249: 1421–7.

80. Hackett ES, Bruemmer J, Hendrickson DA, et al. Buccal mucosal urethroplasty for treatment of recurrent hemospermia in a stallion. J Am Vet Med Assoc 2009;235:1212–5.

81. Sancler-Silva YFR, Silva-Junior ER, Fedorka CE, et al. New treatment for urethral rent in stallions. J Equine Vet Sci 2018;64:89–95.

82. Kilcoyne I, Dechant JE. Complications associated with perineal urethrotomy in 27 equids. Vet Surg 2014;3:691–6.